Praise for *Medico-Legal Issues in Emergency Medicine and*

Overseas Endorsements

I am very impressed with this book. It provides the everyday emergency physician with the tools and understanding of what "rapid medicine" can lead to. Although as emergency physicians we are constantly on our feet and treating patients in a race against time, we have to do it with compassion for both patients and their families. I will definitively recommend this book to all of my residents and graduates. Thank you for putting a lot of complex information into accessible and easy-to-understand material.

Juan F Acosta, DO, FACOEP, FACEP
Assistant Clinical Professor
Weill Cornell Medical College
Program Director, Emergency Medicine Residency
Research Director
Medical Director of Pre-hospital Care
St Barnabas Hospital, Bronx, New York
USA

It is a rare privilege to be able to write an endorsement for a book. It is even rarer to be privileged to write an endorsement for a priceless book. It is refreshing to know that despite the physical boundaries between Singapore and the Philippines, the ethical dilemmas faced by emergency physicians practising in both countries are similar. This book gives practical and timely insights on handling difficult cases in the Emergency Department. From child abuse to advance directives, difficult relatives, and issues on disclosure and non-disclosure, the emergency physician will definitely be able to relate to the vignettes given in the book. Allowing a lawyer and a clinician who encounter these problems on a day-to-day basis to write as a team was a wonderful strategy. I specially enjoyed the take-home messages from each case. Congratulations to both authors for a job well done!

Victoria Cabrera-Ribaya, **MD**
Pediatric Emergency Medicine
Department Chair
Department of Emergency Medicine
St Luke's Medical Center
Philippines

This book is a long-awaited medico-legal guide for those practising in emergency departments. The 35 scenarios essentially cover most of the dilemmas facing emergency physicians in their daily practice, explaining in detail the steps to tackle conflicts between the good faith of the doctor and the right of autonomy of the patient. Even though there is a strong Singaporean flavour, the broad principles apply generally to our increasingly litigious society. The book is well written and enjoyable.

Dr Chung Chin Hung

Chief of Service, Accident & Emergency Department
North District Hospital, Hong Kong
Editor-in-chief, Hong Kong Journal of Emergency Medicine

Professors Tay and Ooi have done an excellent job of capturing the essence of an extremely important topic, Patient and Physician Medico-legal Rights in the Practice of Emergency Medicine and Family Practice. Using a case-based approach, the authors explore a variety of clinical scenarios which are frequently encountered in the medical practice of these two disciplines. Tough questions such as informed consent, organ donor issues, patient privacy, disclosure and the establishment of a physician-patient relationship are explored in a case-based format which is intuitive, fun and educational. Physicians in emergency departments and in office-based practices would enjoy this excellent book and learn from the wisdom of this attorney-physician writing team.

W Brian Gibler, MD

Professor and Chairman
Department of Emergency Medicine
University of Cincinnati College of Medicine
Cincinnati, Ohio
USA

Readers are certain to learn a great deal about a neglected area of medical practice. The authoritative authors have used a presentation style that emphasizes the high clinical relevance of their material.

Dr Gordon Guyatt

Professor of Medicine and Clinical Epidemiology and Biostatistics
McMaster University
Hamilton, Ontario
Canada

This book provides a very useful and clinically relevant series of case-based emergency scenarios illustrating challenging medico-legal issues. The discussion questions and take-home messages allow the reader to quickly access the most important information. While most relevant to the learners and practitioners of emergency medicine in Singapore, this book is also a useful resource for emergency medicine internationally.

Congratulations to Professors Catherine Tay and Shirley Ooi on the publication of this excellent book.

__Brian R Holroyd__
MD, FACEP, FRCPC
Professor and Chair, Department of Emergency Medicine
Faculty of Medicine and Dentistry
University of Alberta
Canada

My congratulations to both authors for making the effort in producing this valuable and important book in medico-legal issues especially for emergency medical practitioners and general practitioners. Most doctors who work in emergency departments are left in the dark regarding medico-legal issues since there are not many books written pertaining to this issue that can serve as a quick guide and handy reference when they carry out their duties. This may lead them into making a decision or committing a practice that might eventually prove to be inaccurate or have litigation consequences.

Even though this book is written based on Singapore experience, the general rules should be applicable to all of us here in Malaysia. Once again, my sincere congratulations to the writers for their tremendous effort.

__Dr Ismail Mohd Saiboon__
Head and Consultant, Department of Emergency Medicine
Hospital Universiti Kebangsaan Malaysia

I find this book an excellent reference on medical issues for clinicians. It provides extremely important guidance for clinical practice, especially in emergency situations in an increasingly litigious society. All doctors should read this book. I would also strongly recommend it to our medical students.

__Professor Dato' Dr Lokman Saim__
Professor of Otorhinolaryngology and Dean of Faculty of Medicine
Universiti Kebangsaan Malaysia

This excellent work produced by Professors Catherine Tay and Shirley Ooi would certainly assist emergency physicians in making decisions when faced with uncertainty in managing patients with potential medico-legal implications. In its presentation and intention, this book reflects throughout a respect for students and clinicians at all levels of training and experience. This work is very valuable indeed, and a very well-done job by the authors.

Dr Nik Hisamuddin Nik Ab Rahman
MBChB (Glasgow), MMed (USM), Clinical Fellow A&E (Edinburgh)
Consultant in Traumatology & Emergency Medicine
Head of Department of Emergency Medicine
School of Medical Sciences
Universiti Sains Malaysia

Doing research in the chaotic environment of the Emergency Department is tough. Getting patients' consent is even tougher. Ethical and medico-legal conflicts often exist. Being an expert in research ethics and medico-legal aspects, Catherine has drawn good illustrations using acute cases. These cases are found in case scenario 17: Research – Informed Consent and case scenario 29: Research – Waiver of Informed Consent. Catherine has also provided further details of research principles in the appendices. The information is crucial for us, the emergency physicians, who would like to conduct a study in the Emergency Department.

Dr Peter Pang
Chairman of EBM Subcommittee
Scientific Affairs
Hong Kong College of Emergency Medicine

We may live in a contentious world, but like a breath of fresh air, the exemplary efforts of both Professors Catherine Tay and Shirley Ooi have articulated the need for good clinical practice and the preservation of medico-legal ethics, which are directed at the nobility of the medical profession.

Maheinthra Kumar Pushpanathan
Marketing Director
Sanofi Aventis (Malaysia) Sdn Bhd

In the Emergency Department, clinicians are not only required to make rapid medical interventions but must also be able to immediately respond to challenging and complex ethical and medical-legal issues. This case-based book provides a succinct and thorough review of how to approach some of the most complex ethical and medical-legal issues in the Emergency Department. The format challenges the reader to make a decision prior to reviewing the answers. The ethical and medical-legal issues in Singapore are different than those in the United States and other parts of the world. Knowledge of the information presented in the book is essential for medical practitioners.

Jeff Schaider, MD
Chairman, Department of Emergency Medicine
Cook County Hospital
Chicago, Illinois
USA

This book would never have been produced if not for the two capable and professional writers on medico-legal matters. I find the book a useful reference on medical ethics and would recommend it to all practising doctors, medical students and medical lecturers.

Dr Wan Zaidah Abdullah
Lecturer and Haematologist
School of Medical Sciences
Universiti Sains Malaysia

This is an impeccable guide for the practising medical profession. The 35 case studies are stimulating to read. This is indeed a revolutionary and effortless way to learn. As a medico-legal practice guide, it is enjoyable to read, not something that one can say about many other textbooks. This excellent book is essential reading for all medico-legal and administrative professionals, and emergency physicians.

Dr Eddie Yuen
Associate Consultant
Emergency Department, Queen Elizabeth Hospital, Hong Kong
Honorary Clinical Assistant Professor
Accident and Emergency Medicine Academic Unit
The Chinese University of Hong Kong

Local Endorsements

This work by Professors Catherine Tay and Shirley Ooi provides a wealth of useful material for all emergency medicine practitioners who want to provide the best standard of care in an environment of patient and public safety. The examples quoted offer abundant resources for the practice of good patient-oriented emergency medicine in all our communities.

This book is a must for all emergency medicine practitioners.

Clinical Professor V Anantharaman
Chairman
Ministry of Health Emergency Medicine Services Committee
Singapore

This carefully researched, well-written and easy-to-read book will give readers a good understanding of the essential medico-legal principles applicable to commonly encountered scenarios in emergency medicine and general practice. It is full of useful tips and take-home messages, and is a must-read for every physician and medical student.

Associate Professor Au Eong Kah Guan
MBBS, MMed(Ophth), FRCS(Edin), FRCS(Glasg), DRCOphth(Lond), FAMS(Ophth)
Head and Senior Consultant, Department of Ophthalmology and
Visual Sciences, Alexandra Hospital and Jurong Medical Centre, Singapore
Adjunct Associate Professor, Department of Ophthalmology, Yong Loo Lin School of Medicine
National University of Singapore, Singapore
Deputy Director (Research), The Eye Institute, National Healthcare Group, Singapore
Visiting Consultant, Department of Ophthalmology, Tan Tock Seng Hospital, Singapore

The good practice of medicine is based on sound knowledge, judgement, common sense and observance of the law. This book is an invaluable aid to all medical practitioners as it focuses on situations and scenarios that can be real problems when faced at our workplaces – the consultation room and operating table. The take-home messages are simple yet unequivocal – ignorance of the law is no excuse in the highly litigious society of today. Just to quote an already familiar phrase, "Don't leave home without it!"

Dr Chang Tou Liang
MBBS, MMed (Family Medicine), MCFP (Singapore)
Family Physician

This book provides an in-depth look into the many different interesting albeit difficult scenarios that may confront any clinician in Singapore today. I find the concise take-home messages especially useful and easy to follow.

Dr Bobby Cheng Ching Li
Consultant Ophthalmic Surgeon
Singapore National Eye Centre

The Emergency Room is one place that puts the healthcare provider at a disadvantage: not only is the doctor faced with a patient that may not be lucid enough to give a proper history or cooperate with the physical examination, he or she also has to deal with the limitations of time, scarce resources, high emotions of the relatives, and fatigue from the numerous cases and rushing around. He or she has to make a decision in that short period of time and yet, exercise acumen and instinct. I remember my A&E posting in Toa Payoh Hospital; it was filled with trauma and drama, and the many subpoenas that came after that. As the saying goes, "Six months of A&E, six years of Court".

This book is both timely and useful. The cases are both real and relevant. The breadth of the cases cited will serve well to help those faced with similar situations and to avoid being dragged down. This is one book you cannot put down until you are through reading all the cases and the legal advice that follows. The authors are to be congratulated for putting together such a compendium to the emergency medicine handbook that we are used to carrying.

A must-have book to avoid a mishap.

Dr Chin Chong Min
Visiting Consultant Urologist
National University Hospital
Singapore

The choice of appropriate local scenarios and clear, concise responses makes it a handy and practical guide – for healthcare professionals working in both emergency and non-emergency settings. Indeed a timely and commendable effort!

Mr Chua Song Khim
CEO, National University Hospital
Singapore

Professors Catherine Tay and Shirley Ooi have written a concise guide to negotiating the medico-legal pitfalls that we encounter on a daily basis in providing basic and specialist medical care in Singapore. This guide will prove useful to both physicians (in identifying medico-ethical issues as and when they arise) and patients (in being educated on how the law protects their rights and interests in Singapore). It is written in a reader-friendly format of multiple-case scenarios that allows readers to digest the concepts and extrapolate the judgements to future cases they may encounter. This handbook is essential reading for the practising physician involved in patient contact, and is a timely addition to fill the void in layman legal education in Singapore.

Dr E-Shawn Goh
Registrar, Department of Ophthalmology, Tan Tock Seng Hospital
Clinical Tutor, Yong Loo Lin School of Medicine, National University of Singapore

I found the book an interesting read, as it dealt with scenarios commonly encountered in the Emergency Department. Some of the patients we encounter have impaired judgement, and cannot be counted on to make a reasoned decision. This book helps us to traverse around the many pitfalls that we often encounter, and points us in the right direction to seek legal advice. It also makes us aware of the rights of patients, doctors, nurses as well as the relatives. All in all, it is an easy-to-digest gem of a book.

Dr Goh Siang Hiong
Head and Senior Consultant, Department of Emergency Medicine
Changi General Hospital, Singapore
President, Society for Emergency Medicine in Singapore

An interesting and informative book for the medical practitioner. It is especially useful in the context of the changing medico-legal scenario in Singapore. Easy reading, just perfect for the busy medical practitioner!

Dr Leo Seo Wei
Consultant, General Ophthalmology
Acting Head, Paediatric Ophthalmology & Strabismus
The Eye Institute @ Tan Tock Seng Hospital
Visiting Consultant, KK Women's and Children's Hospital

The book offers a clear, concise and to-the-point analysis of issues faced by the practising doctor. The case scenarios are wide ranging and realistic. It is evident that the authors have put together their wealth of experience to produce a most remarkable book. Any practising doctor would do well to read it.

Dr Hoh Sek Tien

MBBS (S'pore), FRCS (Ed), FAMS (Ophth)
Consultant Ophthalmic Surgeon, Glaucoma Service, Singapore National Eye Centre
Adjunct Research Fellow, Singapore Eye Research Institute
Clinical Teacher, Yong Loo Lin School of Medicine, National University of Singapore

This book is jointly written by an emergency physician and an academic lawyer, both of whom have a strong interest in medico-legal issues.

The book contains many medico-legal case studies commonly encountered in the Emergency Department. The case studies, which are explained in a clear and concise manner, will be of relevance to both professionals and lay persons.

Clinical Associate Professor Lim Swee Han

Head and Senior Consultant
Department of Emergency Medicine
Singapore General Hospital

My heartfelt congratulations to Professors Catherine Tay and Shirley Ooi for pooling their brains together to produce this compact, precise and easy-to-understand book. This marvellous masterpiece on medical scenarios encountered in emergency medicine and family practice is very timely, as it succinctly analyses the essential ingredients of medico-legal problems faced by the community with special emphasis on problem-solving skills. It deserves a special place on the bookshelves of doctors, medical students, nurses, attorneys and all those who are involved or interested in this field.

Dr V P Nair

Senior Consultant Cardiologist
Mount Elizabeth Medical Centre
Singapore

A concise and compact reference for the clinician on local medico-legal matters. With greater awareness and a more litigious spirit among patients today, a sound understanding and appreciation of medico-legal matters grows ever more important for the clinician managing patients and their expectations.

The book is neatly and simply organized into short case scenarios with important questions raised and answered. A welcomed handbook for the front-line clinician in Singapore today.

Dr Ng Kee Chong
Head and Senior Consultant
Department of Emergency Medicine
KK Women's and Children's Hospital
Singapore

This is an excellent must-read book that all practitioners should have as a guide. The case scenarios are truly getting more common in our hospitals. While we provide good care to our patients, we should be mindful of the medico-legal challenges in our practice.

Dr Alex Su
Consultant and Head, Emergency Services
Institute of Mental Health
Singapore

A practical reference book for every household, as well as an informative and legally upright publication, explaining the responsible course of action for common medical scenarios.

Agnes Tan Noy Kheng and *Mitchell P Yukon*
Singapore

I found the book to be well written; it conveys both important and concise concepts for medical students and physicians. It should be a recommended read for busy modern-day practitioners to equip themselves with the necessary knowledge to meet the challenges of practising modern emergency medicine safely.

Dr Wilfred Tang
Head, Optometry Centre and Course Chairman
Singapore Polytechnic

This well-written compilation of medico-legal case scenarios serves as an excellent education platform for students and practitioners of medicine and law. It provides invaluable insights into avoiding medical negligence, handling legal and ethical dilemmas, and reducing the various adverse incidents. Overall, it promotes a safer clinical practice and provides a great prophylaxis against medico-legal challenges. I congratulate Catherine and Shirley on their excellent work.

Dr Tien Sim Leng
Senior Consultant Haematologist
Singapore General Hospital

Professors Catherine Tay and Shirley Ooi have written an excellent guide to navigating the complex legal terrain of the modern practice of medicine. This new book, the first of its kind in Singapore, will be a helpful resource for students of medicine and law, doctors, lawyers and the general public. With clear examples and memorable lessons to be learned from each example, Professors Tay and Ooi use their engaging teaching skills to enlighten all of us about this challenging and timely topic.

Professor John Wong
Dean, Yong Loo Lin School of Medicine
National University of Singapore

With an increasingly litigious society, the medical profession is challenged with potential medico-legal controversies and implications. The authors have succinctly and concisely brought together a number of relevant case scenarios to illustrate various medico-legal problems in the clinical management of common medical conditions. The take-home messages at the end of each case are particularly useful summaries of important learning points to be remembered.

This is an excellent and practical book that covers the topic well, with good explanations and learning points for the medical profession.

Dr Yip Chee Chew
Consultant and Eye Surgeon
Department of Ophthalmology and Visual Sciences
Alexandra Hospital
Singapore

Medico-Legal Issues in Emergency Medicine and Family Practice

Case Scenarios

Catherine Tay

Shirley Ooi

Singapore • Boston • Burr Ridge, IL • Dubuque, IA • Madison, WI • New York • San Francisco
St. Louis • Bangkok • Kuala Lumpur • Lisbon • London • Madrid • Mexico City
Milan • Montreal • New Delhi • Seoul • Sydney • Taipei • Toronto

The *McGraw·Hill* Companies

Medico-Legal Issues in Emergency Medicine and Family Practice
Case Scenarios

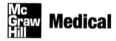 **Medical**

This book intends to highlight some medico-legal issues in common scenarios in emergency medicine and family practice. It is not intended for use as a medical reference guide. It is not a substitute for your lawyers whom you should consult.

1 2 3 4 5 6 7 8 9 10 CTF BJE 20 09 08

When ordering this title, use **ISBN 978-007-126553-9** or **MHID 007-126553-8**

Printed in Singapore

To my uncle, Emeritus Professor Wong Hock Boon, the Father of Paediatrics

Catherine Tay

To God, the source of all human wisdom, insight and understanding
and
To all the past and present doctors of NUH EMD who have co-laboured with me to serve our patients

Shirley Ooi

Foreword I

This is a timely and concise publication which has been written in a very practical scenario-based format. The authors have chosen common clinical settings that may confront the practising clinician in the emergency department of a hospital but the principles may well apply in primary care or in the acute admission wards of hospitals.

As busy medical practitioners, we are concerned with the medical care of patients and should always seek to deliver the most appropriate care. At the same time, doctors should be aware of the law pertaining to the care of their patients and particularly the situation in Singapore at which this book is addressed.

I believe this joint effort between an emergency medicine specialist and a lawyer with an interest in medico-legal matters will address an important gap in our available literature. Its local context should make the book relevant reading and the style of presentation should certainly make it pleasant to read as well.

Associate Professor Benjamin Ong
Senior Consultant, Division of Neurology
Chairman, Medical Board
National University Hospital
Associate Professor, Department of Medicine
Yong Loo Lin School of Medicine
National University of Singapore

Foreword II

My father, who was an ophthalmic surgeon, told me once when I was a trainee, that if a surgeon said that he had never made a mistake, then either he had not done enough surgery or he was not telling the truth. I think the same can apply to emergency physicians who face the threat of complaints or litigation. In a world of increasing litigations, we need to be careful in what we do, think and record, and how we communicate. It is ideal that we do not make mistakes, but if a mistake is made, we should learn lessons from it. Having practised emergency medicine for the last 35 years, I have realized the importance of confidentiality, data protection and communication. Professors Catherine Tay and Shirley Ooi bring with them vast experience from teaching at the Business School and practising emergency medicine, respectively, in writing this book. Its 35 case scenarios provide enough material on the various aspects of medico-legal issues that we may face working in the Emergency Department. The book, with its question-and-answer format, is easy to read and follow. No one can ever provide all the answers for every eventuality or possible pitfall. This book does not claim that either; it provides a common-sensical approach and thinking process. I hope those who use this book will find it as useful as I do.

Dr Gautam G Bodiwala
CBE, DL, DSc (Hon), MS, FRCSEd, FRCP, FCEM, FIFEM
Consultant in Emergency Medicine
Founding President, Medico-Legal Society in Leicestershire
United Kingdom

Foreword III

It was a pleasure to go through the manuscript of this book which deals with many well-thought out case scenarios, on matters which could confront and confound many general practitioners and doctors of various levels in the accident and emergency departments of hospitals.

Professors Catherine Tay and Shirley Ooi are to be congratulated for their splendid efforts in conceiving this book. They have performed invaluable public service in assisting the front-line doctors who have to deal with urgent or emergency cases, often involving strong emotions on the part of the relatives or friends who have brought the patient along. This is because in these people's subjective judgement, immediate and preferential attention is required, and any doctor who does not dance to that tune, is to be viewed as a detestable public enemy.

This book would also be most useful to interested laymen, and to law students and lawyers alike who may wish to enter into the difficult world of medical ethics and medical treatment and diagnosis.

I am happy to recommend this book as good and useful reading to all concerned, coupled with the caveat that the value of a book cannot be judged by its size or weight.

Dr Myint Soe, PBM
MA, PhD (Cambridge), MA (Illinois)
BA (Rangoon), Barrister-at-law
Advocate and Solicitor
Singapore

Preface

Both authors met in class at the National University Hospital (NUH), Singapore, when Professor Shirley Ooi was teaching evidence-based medicine to Year 3 National University of Singapore (NUS) medical students in 2000. In 2001, Professors Shirley Ooi and Catherine Tay decided to collaborate in writing this book, which is long overdue, as both of them have been conducting the medico-legal forum at the Emergency Medicine Department (EMD) in NUH every six months for each new batch of medical officers. Many of the case scenarios cited in the book are the ones they have used in their biannual teaching in the NUH EMD, but many more new ones have been added specifically for this book.

Ethics, law and professionalism, including medicine and society, are crucial in the practice of medicine and surgery. This is reflected in the new curriculum of the Yong Loo Lin School of Medicine at NUS, where these topics are an integral part of the five years of medical school studies, from the first year into the final academic year.

This book, the first of its kind in Singapore, presents a series of case scenarios commonly faced in the Emergency Department (ED) of any hospital. This is a high risk area for medico-legal issues with increasing complaints by patients and their relatives. There are also some scenarios that may be encountered by general practitioners.

This book, which is aimed at ED doctors, medical and law students, and general practitioners, is written in a simple and clear language. However, patients and the general reader may also benefit in knowing their rights at the ED.

The authors would like to thank Associate Professor Benjamin Ong, Dr Gautam G Bodiwala and Dr Myint Soe for writing the Forewords. We would also like to thank everyone who wrote the endorsements for this book.

A very special thank you to Dr Albert Myint Soe from Myint Soe & Selvaraj who spent many hours and weekends poring over the manuscript of this book, reviewing it thoroughly and giving many valuable comments.

Many thanks go to Dr Leo Seo Wei, consultant ophthalmologist from Tan Tock Seng Hospital, for contributing ophthalmology case scenarios 33 and 34 and Dr E-Shawn Goh, registrar at the Department of Opthalmology, Tan Tock Seng Hospital and clinical tutor at the Department of Ophthalmology, Yong Loo Lin School of Medicine, NUS, for contributing ophthalmology case scenarios 31 and 32.

A big thank you to Dr Amila Punyadasa, registrar at the NUH Emergency Medicine Department for reading through the manuscript and pointing out our typographical errors. The authors would also like to acknowledge Mr Edmund Kronenburg, director and head of litigation at the Tan Peng Chin LLC for discussing many of these case scenarios with them during the six-monthly medico-legal forum in NUH. Thanks also go to Daniel Atticus Xu, advocate and solicitor from Myint Soe & Selvaraj, for his invaluable comments on case scenario 5.

The authors welcome any feedback or queries on new scenarios. You may e-mail them at tayooi@yahoo.com.

The law is stated as at August 2007.

Catherine Tay Swee Kian
Bachelor of Laws (Hons) (Queen Mary College, University of London);
Master of Laws (Queen Mary College, University of London);
Barrister-at-Law (Lincoln's Inn, England);
Advocate & Solicitor (Singapore);
Associate Professor, Department of Business Policy, NUS Business School,
National University of Singapore

Shirley Ooi Beng Suat
MBBS (Singapore), FRCSEd (A&E), FAMS;
Chief and Senior Consultant Emergency Physician,
Emergency Medicine Department,
National University Hospital, Singapore;
Clinical Associate Professor at the Yong Loo Lin School of Medicine,
National University of Singapore;
Adjunct Professor, Department of Emergency Medicine,
Universiti Kebangsaan Malaysia

August 2007

About the Authors

Catherine Tay Swee Kian is an associate professor lecturing law at the Department of Business Policy, NUS Business School, National University of Singapore (NUS). Prof Tay also lectures on medical law and biomedical ethics in the NUS Faculty of Dentistry in the Graduate Programme Management in Law and the Practice of Dentistry and Ethics. She has supervised medical students in the legal aspects of medical practice in the Special Study Module at the NUS Faculty of Medicine. She also supervises year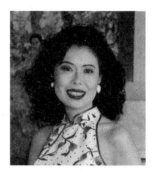
4 medical students at the Yong Loo Lin School of Medicine, NUS, in medico-legal and business issues in their electives. Prof Tay is an advocate and solicitor of the Supreme Court of Singapore, and a barrister-at-law (of Lincoln's Inn, United Kingdom). She is the author of 28 law books.

Prof Tay is a member of the Institutional Review Board of SingHealth Polyclinics, and a member of the National Healthcare Group (NHG) Domain Specific Review Board tasked to review the scientific and ethical aspects of research protocols. A former member of the Research and Ethics Committee of Alexandra Hospital, Prof Tay was also the medical-legal adviser to the Institute of Mental Health/Woodbridge Hospital.

Prof Tay studied law at Queen Mary College, University of London, and graduated with a Bachelor of Laws with Honours in 1977 and a Master of Laws in 1979, specializing in company, shipping, insurance and marine insurance laws. She was called to the English Bar by Lincoln's Inn in 1978. She did her pupillage under the Honourable Lady Mary Hogg in London before returning to Singapore to join the law firm of Rodyk & Davidson.

Prof Tay won the Aw Boon Haw and Aw Boon Par Memorial Prize for the overall best student in 1980 during her postgraduate practical law course in Singapore. She was called to the Singapore Bar in 1980.

In February 1984 and July 1986, Prof Tay made representations to the Parliamentary Select Committee on the recent Companies (Amendment) Bills 1984 and 1986.

Prof Tay's books include

- *Slim Chance Fat Hope* (2004, World Scientific Publishing)
- *Infectious Diseases Law and SARS* (2003, Times Books International)

- *How to Write a Will?* (2003, Big Publications Pte Ltd)
- *Medical Negligence* (2001, Times Books International)
- *Resolving Disputes by Arbitration* (1998, Singapore University Press)
- *A Guide to Protecting Your Ideas, Inventions, Trade Marks and Products* (1997, Times Books International)
- *Copyright and the Protection of Designs* (1997, SNP Publishers Pte Ltd)
- *Buying and Selling Your Property: An Essential Guide to the Singapore Property Market* (1994, Times Books International)
- *Contract Law including E-Commerce Law* (1987, Times Books International)
- *Your Rights as a Consumer: A Guide to Sale of Goods, Hire-Purchase and Small Claims Tribunal* (1986, Times Books International)
- *Directors' Duties and Liabilities including Insider Trading* (1985, Times Books International)
- *Bankruptcy: The Law and Practice* (1984, Butterworths)

Prof Tay has published numerous articles in international peer reviewed journals, such as *BIOETHICS, Hong Kong Journal of Emergency Medicine,* (United Kingdom) *Journal of Business Law,* (United Kingdom) *Business Law Review,* (United Kingdom) *The Company Lawyer,* (United Kingdom) *Insolvency Law & Practice,* (United Kingdom) *Tolley's Professional Negligence,* (United Kingdom) *Tottel's Professional Negligence,* the *Singapore Dental Journal,* the *APLAR Journal of Rheumatology,* the *Malayan Law Journal,* the *Securities Industry Review* and *The Singapore Law Gazette.*

Prof Tay was a member of the editorial board of the *Singapore Accountant Journal, Journal of the Institute of Certified Public Accountants of Singapore* and (United Kingdom) *The Company Lawyer.* She sat on the board of overseas editors for the (United Kingdom) *Journal of Financial Crime,* an official publication of the Cambridge International Symposium on Economic Crime. She has presented papers at many conferences and seminars on business law, medical law, and company and insolvency laws both overseas and in Singapore. Prof Tay is an examiner on law subjects for a number of professional bodies in Singapore and overseas.

Prof Tay lectures on medical law and biomedical ethics at the Singapore General Hospital, National Heart Centre, National Skin Centre, National Healthcare Group College, Changi General Hospital, Toa Payoh Hospital, Alexandra Hospital, National University Hospital, Mount Elizabeth Hospital, Department of Anatomy of the Yong Loo Lin School of Medicine, NUS, Singapore Dental Association and SingHealth Polyclinics in Tampines, Bedok and Marine Parade. In March 2003, she was invited to speak at the Third ASEAN Conference in Primary Health Care organized by the Perak Medical Practitioners Society in Ipoh, Malaysia.

She was an invited conference speaker on "Ethical Issues on Embryonic Human Stem Cell Research and Therapeutic Cloning" at a life sciences conference organized by the Indian Medical Council of Research in Mumbai, India, in September 2006.

Prof Tay also lectures on "Medical Ethics of Informed Consent" in the Singapore Good Clinical Practice Programme – Basic GCP (Clinical Trials Management Course) organized by the Yong Loo Lin School of Medicine, NUS. Prof Tay was the supervisor of the medical student who won the Medical Student Award in the Special Study Module 2001 at the Yong Loo Lin School of Medicine for the topic on "Genetics, Privacy and the Law".

A poster co-authored by Prof Tay and Assoc Prof (Dr) Giam Yoke Chin, a National Skin Centre senior consultant dermatologist, won the Best Poster Award in the Allied Sciences Section during the National Healthcare Group (NHG) Annual Scientific Congress 2004. The abstract has been published in a supplement issue of *Annals*, a peer-reviewed and indexed medical journal published by the Academy of Medicine, Singapore.

Prof Tay is a legal consultant who has appeared on many television segments produced by the then Television Corporation of Singapore. She has spoken on legal subjects on MediaCorp's radio programmes and co-hosted a weekly talk show "In the Eyes of the Law" on NTUC's RadioHeart. Prof Tay was a consultant to the MediaCorp television series on consumer laws, "What's Your Case", which was shown on Channel 5.

Prof Tay participates actively in many professional and charitable organizations for which she has received several titles and awards. She was a committee member of the Advice and Referral Service in the Singapore Council of Women's Organizations. In 1990–2000, she was the president of the Business and Professional Women's Association, Singapore. In March 1992, she was a nominee for the Woman of the Year Award. In May 1994 Prof Tay received the Paul Harris Fellow Award from Rotary International in recognition of her community service.

Selected Peer-reviewed Journal Articles Publications

1. Medical Ethics of Informed Consent: A Survey of Medical Professionals in Singapore, with Dr Giam Yoke Chin, Dr EST Tan, Dr M Chio, Dr Goh Chee Leok and YH Chan, (United Kingdom) *Tottel's Journal of Professional Negligence*, December 2006, Vol. 22, No. 4, pages 236–250.
2. New Developments in Competition Law in Singapore, (United Kingdom) *Business Law Review*, May 2006, Vol. 27, No. 5, pages 120–125.

3. Recent Developments in Informed Consent: The Basis of Modern Medical Ethics, *APLAR Journal of Rheumatology*, December 2005, pages 165–170, Asia Pacific League of Associations for Rheumatology.

4. New Developments in Duty of Care: The Singapore Approach to Negligence in Product Liability after the Slim 10 case, (United Kingdom) *Business Law Review*, May 2005, pages 116–124.

5. Biomedical Technology in Progress with Responsibility, *BIOETHICS*, June 2005, Vol. 19, No. 3, pages 290–303.

6. Professional Negligence and Medical Professional Privilege: Impact of D v Kong Sim Guan, (United Kingdom) *Tolley's Journal of Professional Negligence*, 2004, Vol. 20, No.1, pages 33–40.

7. Infectious Diseases Law and Severe Acute Respiratory Syndrome: Medical and Legal Responses and Implications: The Singapore Experience, (Australia) *APLAR Journal of Rheumatology*, 2004, Vol. 7, No. 2, pages 123–129, Asia Pacific League of Associations for Rheumatology.

8. Understanding the Basic Elements of Informed Consent: A Survey of Medical Professionals, supplement issue of *Annals*, October 2004, page S93, Academy of Medicine.

9. Biomedical Technology in Progress with Responsibility: An Ethical Legal Social Review of Human Stem Cell Research, Therapeutic and Reproductive Cloning in Singapore, supplement issue of *Annals*, October 2004, page S140, Academy of Medicine.

10. Is There a Doctor on Board? Medical Liability During In-flight Emergencies, with Dr F Lateef and Dr N Nimbkar, *Hong Kong Journal of Emergency Medicine*, July 2003, Vol. 10, No. 3, pages 191–198.

11. Standard of Dental Care: Ambit of the Bolam Test, *Singapore Dental Journal*, July 2003, Vol. 25, No. 1, pages 1–2.

12. Interpretation of the Bolam Test in the Standard of Medical Care: Impact of the Gunapathy Case and Beyond, (United Kingdom) *Tolley's Journal of Professional Negligence*, 2003, Vol. 19, No. 2, pages 384–394.

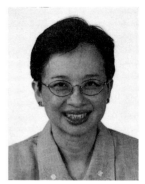

Shirley Ooi Beng Suat was a former ASEAN pre-university scholar from Penang, Malaysia, and a Singapore Public Service Commission Local Merit Scholarship holder for medicine in the National University of Singapore (NUS). She obtained her FRCSEd (A&E) in 1992, and became a Fellow of the Academy of Medicine, Singapore, in 1998. She worked in Edinburgh, UK, in 1992 and did a Trauma Fellowship in the University of Cincinnati Medical Center, USA, from October 1996 to June 1997. Since July 2006, Prof Ooi has been Chief of the Emergency Medicine Department (EMD) at the National University Hospital (NUH). She has been a clinical associate professor at the Yong Loo Lin School of Medicine, NUS, since 2004 and an adjunct professor at the Department of Emergency Medicine, Universiti Kebangsaan Malaysia since 2007.

Prof Ooi, whose passion is in teaching and mentoring, has been invited to give multiple lectures locally and overseas. She was the Department Director of Postgraduate Education at the NUH EMD from 1997 to 2006. Prof Ooi received the NUH Postgraduate Teaching Excellence Award in 2002, and the FY 04 HMDP award to do the American College of Emergency Physicians (ACEP) Teaching Fellowship Program in Dallas, Texas in 2004–2005. Prof Ooi is currently a member of the Specialist Training Committee in Emergency Medicine and chairing the National Combined Advance Specialist Training Committee for Emergency Medicine. She is also in the management committee of the Chapter of Emergency Physicians, Academy of Medicine, Singapore and the Society for Emergency Medicine in Singapore. A facilitator in local and international Evidence-based Medicine (EBM) workshops for many years, she is also chairing the NUH EBM Committee and the Sixth Asia-Pacific EBM workshop to be held in 2008. The book *Guide to the Essentials in Emergency Medicine*, which she co-edited with Clinical Associate Professor Peter Manning and published by McGraw-Hill in 2004, has sold close to 6,000 copies worldwide and gone into its sixth print run.

Prof Ooi has been the Department Director of Research at the NUH EMD since 2003. Her research interest is in emergency cardiac care, especially in studies dealing with the diagnosis of acute myocardial infarction using cardiac biomarkers and electrocardiogram. For the above, she won the 1997 ACEP Research Forum Young Investigator Award for excellence in research and presentation by the Emergency Medicine Foundation, USA. She also won the Best Medical Paper Award at the Society for Emergency Medicine in Singapore Fourth Annual Scientific Meeting in 2003, and an award for being the best oral presenter at one of the free paper sessions during the Third Asian Conference on Emergency Medicine in Hong Kong in October 2004. She has received multiple research grants and published many articles in peer-reviewed journals. She has also contributed multiple book chapters in local and overseas Emergency Medicine textbooks. Currently an associate editor with the *Singapore Medical Journal*, she was given the Singapore Medical Journal 2005 recognition award for reviewing with distinction. She is also a reviewer with the *Annals of the Academy of Medicine of Singapore*. She is actively involved in the organization of Emergency Medicine conferences and scientific meetings.

She is a member of the Joint Final MRCSEd (A&E)/MMed (Emergency Medicine) examination committee as well as an examiner. She has also been invited as an external examiner for the Master of Medicine (Emergency Medicine) organized by Universiti Sains Malaysia, Kota Bahru, Malaysia, in November 2005 and May 2006. Her biography has been selected for inclusion in the sixth edition (2006–2007) of *Marquis Who's Who in Medicine and Healthcare*, the first edition of *Marquis Who's Who in Asia 2007* and the 25th (silver anniversary) edition of *Marquis Who's Who in the World 2008*.

Contents

Case Scenario 1

Drug Overdose – Process of Discharge Against Medical Advice

A 30-year-old female overdoses on 40 tablets of paracetamol. She is brought into the Emergency Department by her husband. She refuses medical treatment and wants to be discharged from the hospital's Emergency Department.

(a) Can a patient who looks alert be allowed to sign a discharge form against the doctor's advice?

(b) If not, should the husband of the patient be allowed to sign on her behalf?

(c) What should the emergency physician do in such a case?

(d) Will the doctor be liable if a suicidal patient is sent home and subsequently commits suicide?

(e) What is involved in the process of discharge against medical advice?

(f) If the patient in the above scenario had overdosed on ten 5 mg tablets of valium and was a little drowsy but still arousable, would your answers to the first four questions still be the same?

Answers

(a) Can a patient who looks alert be allowed to sign a discharge form against the doctor's advice?

No. Alertness is not the touchstone; "competency" is, i.e. the legal capacity of a person to make a considered decision.

In this particular situation, one needs to assess the patient's competency to refuse treatment. Only competent patients can exercise patient autonomy. If a patient is found to be anything but competent, and has no parent (if the patient is below the age of 21 years), legal guardian or representative to speak on her behalf (not a husband, son or sibling, but a court-appointed representative), the doctor cannot allow her to refuse treatment; the doctor must act in the patient's best interests. The doctor's basic duty is to preserve life. The doctor should, however, document in his notes that he cannot determine the patient's competency and until that can be done (e.g. by reference to a psychiatrist), he must presume that the patient is incompetent and act in her best interests.

If, however, the doctor finds the patient to be competent to make the decision whether to refuse or accept treatment, she can lawfully sign the discharge form, even if this is against the best advice of the doctor. However, the doctor should at the bare minimum document that the patient insisted on being discharged against his advice, and that the patient did this despite being fully advised of the risks of refusing treatment.

Documentation or patient charting is very important. If a doctor fails to record an important event in his notes (e.g. his having advised the patient of the risk of refusing treatment), the court will find it very difficult to believe that the event actually occurred.

Anything recorded by the doctor (and his nurses) can also be used as evidence should there be a lawsuit against the doctor. Good notes generally indicate a good quality of medical care. They at least show that you are not a slapdash doctor in terms of keeping patients' records. Clinically, good notes mean that another team of doctors can take over the care of the patient efficiently, in the event that the patient is transferred or in an emergency.

> **Take-home Message**
> Good notes = good defence
> Bad notes = bad defence
> No notes = no defence

(b) If not, should the husband of the patient be allowed to sign on her behalf?

It is a common practice in many medical establishments that a spouse, child or sibling of the patient is allowed to sign a discharge form on the patient's behalf.

In the eyes of the law, however, this act has no real effect. Only the patient herself can consent to being discharged against the advice of a doctor. Only the patient herself can sign a form refusing treatment.

(c) What should the emergency physician do in such a case?

The physician should either ask the patient to sign the form, or if she refuses, act in the patient's best interests and treat her.

However, if the patient wants to sign the form but is unable to do so due to an injury, e.g. an injury to both hands, the discharge form can be signed by someone responsible, such as the patient's close relative or next of kin as a *witness* to the patient's refusal of treatment. This must be clearly documented on the form, e.g. "Signed by MR TAN BOON CHEW, husband of the patient, MDM LEE GEK NEO, witnessing that MDM LEE agrees to the contents of this form and that she wishes to be discharged against the advice of DR GOH KENG WEE". The husband should be asked to hand-write and initial that statement on the discharge form.

(d) Will the doctor be liable if a suicidal patient is sent home and subsequently commits suicide?

Generally speaking, if the doctor did not even address his mind to whether the patient was competent in the circumstances, e.g. he suspected that she might be suicidal but allowed her to sign the discharge form without referring her for psychiatric evaluation, and she dies from the overdose, the doctor will probably be liable.

If he did address his mind to this issue and found her to be competent to refuse treatment, whether he is liable or not will depend on whether he has met the standard of care set out in the *Bolam* test (see Appendix 1 for further details), which, as explained by the *Bolitho* decision, should be responsible, reasonable and respectable (see Appendix 2 for further details). For example: Did the doctor, in adjudging the patient competent, meet the standards expected of any responsible and competent doctor in his shoes? If he did, there is no liability. If he did not (e.g. any responsible and competent doctor would have referred her for psychiatric evaluation), then there is likely to be liability.

Take-home Message

Refer the patient to a specialist, if you need to.
Do what any responsible and competent doctor would do!

(e) What is involved in the process of discharge against medical advice?

Explain to the patient all the risks involved should she refuse treatment, and advise her on whether there are any alternative treatments available. Ask the patient again whether she will agree to medical treatment. Encourage her to discuss her refusal with close relatives or next of kin. (Due to doctor-patient confidentiality, do not do this yourself.) Suggest to the patient that she can contact her family doctor and offer to involve him in her treatment. If she insists on refusing treatment, tell her that she can always change her mind and that she can call you should she want treatment. Document every step in the refusal process. Record in your doctor's notes the names of all witnesses to what you have explained and said to the patient.

Take-home Message

Your longest medical documentation is often when the patient refuses treatment.

(f) **If the patient in the above scenario had overdosed on ten 5 mg tablets of valium and was a little drowsy but still arousable, would your answers to the first four questions still be the same?**

From a medical standpoint, there can no longer be any doubt that the patient is suicidal and incompetent for purposes of refusing treatment. She must be treated even against the protests of close relatives or next of kin. You must act in her best interests until she is in a position to decide whether she requires further medical treatment.

Case Scenario 2

Underage Pregnancy — Concept of "Gillick Competence" and Patient Confidentiality

A 16-year-old schoolgirl is brought in by her teacher to the Emergency Department as she is suspected of being pregnant. A urine pregnancy test confirms that she is pregnant.

(a) What should the doctor do if the girl requests that the doctor withhold the information of her pregnancy from her parents?

(b) Will the consent of the girl's parents be needed if she requests for the termination of her pregnancy?

(c) If the patient in the above scenario had been a 13-year-old schoolgirl, would the answers to the above questions still be the same?

CONTINUED ON

Answers

(a) **What should the doctor do if the girl requests that the doctor withhold the information of her pregnancy from her parents?**

Under the law of confidentiality, every doctor has a duty of confidentiality to his patients. He must keep the medical secrets of his patient.

The duties of patient confidentiality are also found in the codes of medical ethics. The confidentiality of a patient's relationship with his doctor is fundamental to ethical medical practice. The doctor accepts and adopts the fundamental ethical basis of respect for an individual, i.e. autonomy or self-determination and the privacy of the patient. There is a public interest in maintaining that medical confidence. A doctor breaching patient confidentiality may be subject to disciplinary action by the medical profession, apart from possible legal action taken out by the patient.

In the New Zealand case of *Furniss v Fitchett* (1958) NZLR 396, a patient plaintiff successfully sued her doctor in a medical negligence action as she was harmed physically by the doctor's improper disclosure of medical information. The duty of confidentiality is part of the general medical duty of care to the patient.

The ethical duty to maintain patient confidentiality allows patients to disclose information on their health to their doctors freely. Patients are protected from harm that may arise from an unauthorized disclosure of medical information.

The Hippocratic Oath
… Whatever, in connection with my professional service, or not in connection with it, I see or hear, in the life of men, which ought not to be spoken of abroad, I will not divulge, as reckoning that all such should be kept secret.

The Declaration of Geneva
… I will respect the secrets which are confided in me, even after the patient has died.

The Singapore Physician's Pledge
I solemnly pledge to … respect the secrets which are confided in me …

However, there are certain exceptions when the doctor is allowed to reveal a patient's medical information. These are

- when a patient consents to disclosure
- to comply with the statutory duty to report infectious diseases requiring notification, e.g. under the Infectious Diseases Act
- to comply with a court order

- when disclosure is in the public interest, e.g. *W v Egell* (1990) 1 All E.R. 835
- when disclosure can prevent or avert serious harm to a patient
- to communicate with other doctors on treatment

There are circumstances where a girl under the age of 16 may want to keep a medical secret from her parents such as asking for contraceptives from doctors. If the girl is "Gillick competent" (*Gillick v West Norfolk & Wisbech Area Health Authority* (1986) 1 AC 112), i.e. she is competent to make a decision on medical treatment, then the doctor should not involve her parents, since she understands the implications of the choices she makes. Here, the doctor has a duty to promote the girl's best interest as her welfare is very important.

Therefore, if the 16-year-old girl is "Gillick competent" in that she understands the counselling of the doctor, then the doctor should withhold the information from her parents because of the law of confidentiality. If the doctor assesses that the girl cannot understand him, then her parents must be informed.

Take-home Message

It is the doctor's duty to determine whether a patient, who is below the age of 16, is "Gillick competent" and is able to understand him.

(b) Will the consent of the girl's parents be needed if she requests for the termination of her pregnancy?

Under the Termination of Pregnancy Act, a doctor does not require parental consent for teenage abortion. Otherwise, the teenager may

- try dangerous medicines
- experiment with unproven methods
- be driven to unlicensed practitioners
- resort to suicide

There is, however, a structured procedure for teenage abortion. The girl must undergo pre-abortion counselling at a designated counselling centre conducted by trained nurses and medical social workers. The structured abortion counselling aims to educate on issues such as

- responsible love
- sexual behaviour
- contraceptive methods
- psychosocial factors (predisposing girls towards sexual relationships, and to prevent repeat pregnancies)

The counselling sessions will include other options such as

- carrying the foetus to term
- encouragement to confide in parents
- health and safety of teenagers

Under the Termination of Pregnancy Act, the only legal requirement is that the abortion must be performed by a registered medical practitioner with the written consent of the pregnant woman. Parental or guardian consent is not required for a patient below 21 years of age.

Therefore, if the 16-year-old girl requests for the termination of her pregnancy, the doctor need not obtain her parents' consent under the Termination of Pregnancy Act. The doctor must, however, obtain the written consent of the pregnant girl.

Take-home Message

The consent of parents and guardians is not needed in the termination of a pregnancy for persons below 21 years of age.

(c) If the patient in the above scenario had been a 13-year-old schoolgirl, would the answers to the above questions still be the same?

The answers to the first two questions will be the same, except that a statutory rape is involved for persons under 14 years of age. The doctor has a duty to report this matter to the authorities. Sexual intercourse with a girl below 16 years of age is an offence under the Women's Charter.

Case Scenario 3

Self-harm – Concept of Abscondment and "False Imprisonment"

A 15-year-old boy slashes his wrist because of relationship problems. He is brought to the hospital by a friend. He refuses to be admitted or see a psychiatrist, and does not want his parents to know.

(a) What should the emergency physician do?

(b) If the patient turns violent and threatens to kill himself but still refuses to be admitted, can the physician go against his wishes and get him admitted after sedating him?

(c) If the patient escapes (absconds) from the hospital and meets with an accident outside the hospital, will the hospital be liable?

(d) If the above patient had been a 25-year-old man, would the answers to the first two questions still be the same?

Answers

(a) What should the emergency physician do?

He should act in the boy's best interests and treat the boy. If this extends to a psychiatric evaluation, he should proceed to refer the boy. The *Gillick* principle does not allow a minor to *refuse* life-saving medical treatment. The boy's parents should be found and notified. After they arrive, the parents have the right to consent to, or refuse, treatment for their son.

(b) If the patient turns violent and threatens to kill himself but still refuses to be admitted, can the physician go against his wishes and get him admitted after sedating him?

Yes. See answer to (a) above.

(c) If the patient escapes (absconds) from the hospital and meets with an accident outside the hospital, will the hospital be liable?

This depends on how and why the boy absconded. If he did so despite the best measures being put in place, the hospital will not be liable. If the hospital had measures but was substandard in implementing them, the hospital could be found liable.

The *Bolam* test (refer to Appendix 1 for further details) applies here.

Take-home Message

Do what is accepted current practice under the *Bolam* test.
But the practice must be logical under the *Bolitho* case.

(d) If the above patient had been a 25-year-old man, would the answers to the first two questions still be the same?

Yes, except that the man's parents would have no say in his treatment, even if they were to come to the hospital. The doctor would have to act in the man's best interests until he is again able to make decisions for himself, i.e. until he regains competency.

Take-home Message

Be aware of mental health laws.
Ignorance of the law is not a privilege.
It is your misfortune.

Case Scenario 4

Drunken Driving – When to Legally Do an Alcohol Level Test

A 40-year-old motorcyclist is involved in a traffic accident. He is drowsy and incoherent. The police want you to take his blood for an alcohol level test by producing a signed document to say that the patient has agreed to have it done.

(a) What should you do as a doctor?

(b) Can the police insist that the doctor produce an incidental alcohol level taken by him without the patient's consent and use that to charge the patient in court?

(c) Can an alcohol level test be done on any patient without his or her consent?

Answers

(a) What should you do as a doctor?

As an emergency physician, your primary duty remains that of a medical doctor, i.e. to save lives. You should be very careful as the 40-year-old motorcyclist is a patient who is in a very vulnerable state, being under police custody.

The police officers will usually bring such drunk drivers as accused persons to the hospital during the hours of darkness when the Emergency Department is crowded with patients in a more life-threatening condition and the hospital's manpower is scarce. You ought to give the drunk motorcyclist a general examination to see if there are any signs of physical abuse (by the police), then ask the motorcyclist to confirm that he has signed the consent form voluntarily, even if it is in the presence of the junior police officers. You must record down the name, service number and the police station or unit of the police officer who produces the signed document. You must ask yourself whether the motorcyclist is a hospital patient. If so, you exercise control over the situation and manage the patient's needs over and above that of the police.

If the motorcyclist is drunk and drowsy, is in an incoherent state and does not require immediate medical attention, there is no urgency. You may attend to the other patients first, and allow the motorcyclist to become more sober before attempting to ask him whether he has consented to the blood test. The police ought to have conducted the breath analyser test whenever possible.

As a matter of police deployment, the escorting police officer is usually the most junior and the least experienced uniformed officer. If you need any clarification, you may ask to speak to his superior (usually an inspector or station inspector) by calling the police station or unit directly. Such details ought to be available in the accompanying police documents.

(b) Can the police insist that the doctor produce an incidental alcohol level taken by him without the patient's consent and use that to charge the patient in court?

The Road Traffic Act empowers the Deputy Commissioner of Police to direct the medical doctor to produce an incidental alcohol level of the motorcyclist taken by the doctor *only* if there is a road traffic accident between vehicles or involving someone who is injured or has died as a result of the accident, and the motorcyclist is injured to such an extent that he is not able to take a breath analyser test or give his consent.

Further, doctors must observe patient confidentiality even in requests from the police. As it is presumably a piece of paper regarding a test already made by the hospital, it could be regarded as a document or some other thing under section 58(1) of the Criminal Procedure Code (Cap. 68). The police will have to show that it is needed for the purposes of a criminal investigation. There should be a request in writing signed by at least an Inspector of Police.

(c) Can an alcohol level test be done on any patient without his or her consent?

See suggested answer to (b) above. See Appendix 4 for further details.

Case Scenario 5

Drug Abuse – Dilemma of Reporting v Not Reporting

A 20-year-old patient complains of chest pain. On questioning, he admits to taking cocaine regularly.

(a) Should you report him to the authorities?

(b) Will this constitute a breach of confidentiality?

Answers

(a) Should you report him to the authorities?

Yes. Under Regulation 19 of the Misuse of Drugs Regulations 1973, a doctor must report a drug addict within seven days if he considers or has reasonable grounds to suspect that his patient is taking drugs. He should report to the Central Narcotics Bureau as well to the Director of Medical Services.

All public hospitals have a police post run by a junior police officer on different shifts. If a doctor is of the opinion that his patient is taking drugs, he can alert the duty officer at the hospital police post as soon as practicable after rendering medical services to the patient.

(b) Will this constitute a breach of confidentiality?

Yes, this constitutes a breach of confidentiality. However, there are limitations or exceptions to the general duty of medical care to keep a patient's medical information secret. Examples of such exceptions include a patient's consent or public interest. Cocaine is a Class A drug under the Misuse of Drugs Act (Cap. 185).

Case Scenario 6

Withholding of Diagnosis from a Patient – Is It Legal?

You suspect a patient to have liver cancer. However, the patient's relatives refuse to let you reveal the diagnosis to him as they are quite sure that he will not be able to take it as he has a weak heart.

(a) Should you comply with the wishes of your patient's relatives?

(b) Once the diagnosis of liver cancer is confirmed, can the patient sue you for withholding the diagnosis from him?

(c) In the event that you reveal the diagnosis to the patient and he collapses and dies, can you be sued by his relatives?

Answers

(a) Should you comply with the wishes of your patient's relatives?

No. You should not comply with the wishes of the patient's relatives. Your medical duty of care is to the patient himself and not to his relatives. It is a legal duty as well as an ethical duty to keep a patient's medical information private. The patient's relatives should not even be told of the suspected liver cancer without his consent. As a doctor, you would have breached your patient's confidentiality by telling his relatives about the diagnosis without his consent.

The duty of keeping confidence exists in the code of medical ethics. In *Hunter v Mann* (1974) QB 767, the court held that:

> ... the doctor is under a duty not to disclose (voluntarily) without the consent of his patient information which he, the doctor, has obtained in his professional capacity, save in very exceptional circumstances.

The scope of this duty of confidentiality is a mixture of tort (i.e. wrongful actions), contract, equity and property concepts. A doctor's duty is fiduciary based on trust and the patient can sue the doctor for any breach of confidentiality. This was the case in *Furniss v Fitchett* (1958) NZLR 396, where the doctor had been the regular doctor of a man and his wife. When relations between husband and wife were strained, the doctor gave the husband a document containing his medical observations. Later, in a court proceeding on matrimonial matters, the husband's lawyer produced the said document, which caused the wife to suffer a grievous shock that damaged her health. The woman then sued the doctor successfully for damages (i.e. monetary compensation) in a tort claim. The court further held that the showing of the document to the woman by her husband's lawyer was foreseeable by the doctor and was the very thing that the law required the doctor to take care to avoid.

Under the law of negligence, the general duty is not to cause foreseeable harm to one another in situations where the parties have a very close relationship; any unauthorized disclosure of confidential information about a patient is grounds for a negligence lawsuit, if the disclosure causes damage to the patient. But there are certain exceptions where disclosure is allowed such as when a patient consents to it or if it is in the public interest to disclose it.

The medical profession has a strict ethical duty to protect confidential information, as seen in the codes of ethics of the Singapore Medical Association, the Singapore Medical Council and the Singapore Dental Association.

A doctor also cannot reveal a patient's medical information to another doctor unless he is also a doctor in the team directly caring for the patient.

Take-home Message

It is best practice for a doctor to ask a patient for his consent to reveal his medical condition to another specialist doctor for better medical care, and to give the patient the option of objecting to it.

(b) Once the diagnosis of liver cancer is confirmed, can the patient sue you for withholding the diagnosis from him?

Yes, the patient can sue the doctor if he fails to inform the patient of his diagnosis. It is the doctor's legal and ethical duty to inform a patient of his diagnosis. Under the fundamental principles of medical ethics of fidelity, which is truth-telling and confidentiality, and veracity, which is honesty, a doctor is obliged to be honest with his patient and to reveal his diagnosis. Fidelity is the doctor's duty to observe the pledges made by the medical profession to society and to patients.

Take-home Message

A doctor must tell his patient his diagnosis as soon as possible, otherwise the doctor is in breach of his ethical and legal duty.

(c) In the event that you reveal the diagnosis to the patient and he collapses and dies, can you be sued by his relatives?

The relatives cannot have higher rights than the deceased. As the law generally allows full disclosure to the deceased, prima facie (i.e. on the face of it), there is no negligence. There can be negligence in the way or the method used in communicating the information. The patient with liver cancer will also be in a weak state. If he is aroused in a rough manner and unnecessarily robust language is used, which causes the patient to collapse, the doctor concerned and the hospital can be sued for negligence. The damages will be for bereavement, but the loss of future earnings is not recoverable.

The Administrator or Executor (who will be a close relative) can sue on behalf of the estate. It all depends on the totality of the facts involved.

The above is a civil proceeding. However, it is interesting to note that in criminal law, under Section 93 of the Penal Code, should the patient die by the doctor's communication, the doctor is protected should there be a lawsuit initiated by the patient's relatives.

Section 93 of the Penal Code – Communication Made in Good Faith
No communication made in good faith is an offence by reason of any harm to the person to whom it is made, if it is made for the benefit of that person.

Illustration

A, a surgeon, in good faith, communicates to a patient his opinion that he cannot live. The patient dies in consequence of the shock. *A* has committed no offence, though he knew it to be likely that the communication might cause the patient's death.

Take-home Message

Communication made in good faith is not a criminal offence if it is made for that person's benefit. This recognizes the fact that a patient has a right to know even when that communication may cause harm to him.

Emergency Procedure – Difficulty in Obtaining Informed Consent

What should you do if you have difficulty obtaining the consent of a patient for an emergency procedure in the following situations?

(a) When the patient is in a state of alcohol or drug intoxication

(b) When communication is a problem because of language difficulties

(c) When the patient is a minor

Answers

(a) **When the patient is in a state of alcohol or drug intoxication**

Medical treatment can only be given with the consent of a competent patient. However, treatment can also be authorized by the court, a parent or legal guardian. Consent is an ethical principle. A patient has a right to know what medical treatment he is getting. The failure to obtain proper and valid consent from a patient is considered a failure to respect a patient's autonomy, which violates his right to self-determination. Medical law respects autonomy by demanding the consent of a patient.

Justice Cardozo in *Schloendorff v Society of New York Hospital*, 105 NE 92 (NY 1914) said:

> Every human being of adult years and sound mind has a right to determine what shall be done with his own body, and a surgeon who performs an operation without his patient's consent commits an assault, for which he is liable.

Consent must be voluntarily given by a patient with his understanding of the nature, risks, benefits and limitations of the proposed treatment, and any other alternatives or options available. Medical treatment given without "real" consent is grounds for action in trespass for which the patient can sue the doctor for damages. Consent may be given orally or in writing. However, it is the doctor's duty to ensure that a patient understands the information given to him. The best practice here is that of a doctor giving an oral or a written test to his patient.

In an emergency situation where a patient is in a coma or unconscious, a doctor can perform emergency medical treatment without getting the patient's consent because it is based on "implied consent" or the doctrine of necessity to save a life. For a surgical intervention that involves risks, it is advisable to get two consultant physicians to sign on behalf of the incompetent patient. The decision for medical treatment cannot be based on whether it was convenient then to perform the treatment. In the Canadian case of *Malette v Shulman* (1990) 67 DLR (4th) 321, the judge said:

> A doctor is not free to disregard a patient's advance instructions any more than he would be free to disregard instructions given at the time of the emergency.

There is "implied consent" in that a patient would have consented to the medical treatment as it was necessary to save him from serious harm or death.

Therefore, under the defence of necessity or implied consent, if a patient is not competent due to alcohol or drug intoxication, a doctor can perform medical treatment without getting the consent of the patient; he must, however, treat the patient in his best interests.

The Singapore Medical Council (SMC) itself recognizes emergency situations under 4.1.7.2 of the SMC Ethical Code and Ethical Guidelines.

(b) **When communication is a problem because of language difficulties**

The doctor should get an interpreter to assist in obtaining proper consent from the patient. If it is an emergency situation to save a life, then the patient's consent can be waived and the doctor must treat the patient in his best interests, as explained in answer (a) above.

(c) **When the patient is a minor**

If the patient is a minor under 21 years of age, the doctor should get the consent of his parents or legal guardian. If the parents or guardians are not available, then the doctor must treat the minor patient in his best interests, if it is an emergency situation to save a life.

When the consent of a patient's parents or legal guardians is not available, those *in loco parentis* will suffice, e.g. the principal or head of his or her school if the patient is a student. Otherwise, the best interests rule applies, but the wishes of the minor should be heard, even if it is not followed.

Take-home Message

Consent must always be obtained from a patient, unless it is an emergency life-threatening situation; if obtaining the patient's consent is difficult, the doctor should go ahead to treat the patient in his best interests.

Case Scenario 8

Non-accidental Injury – Dilemma of Refusal for Admission

You suspect that a five-year-old child being brought to the Emergency Department for multiple bruises may be a victim of non-accidental injury (NAI). You want to admit the patient as you feel it will be safer for the child while investigations are being carried out.

(a) Should the child's parents refuse to have their child admitted, what can you do?

(b) If the child is taken home and eventually dies, and a post-mortem confirms NAI, will the doctor who allowed the child to be taken home be open to a claim for negligence or malpractice?

Answers

(a) Should the child's parents refuse to have their child admitted, what can you do?

The doctor should still admit the child to hospital if that is in the best interests of the child. It is advisable to seek help from the police as this is judged as a life-threatening situation.

(b) If the child is taken home and eventually dies, and a post-mortem confirms NAI, will the doctor who allowed the child to be taken home be open to a claim for negligence or malpractice?

Yes, the doctor may be deemed negligent in allowing the child to be taken home. The doctor should act in the best interests of the child in his medical treatment of the child. From a practical point of view, a five-year-old child will have to sue through his parents. As the child is brought home by his parents, they may also be liable for negligence and can be added as defendants. In any case, the fixed damages for the death of a child will only be $10,000 under Singapore law. Hence, legal proceedings are unlikely.

Case Scenario 9

Withholding of Life-support Procedures – Concept of "Advance Medical Directive"

An 89-year-old female with severe breathlessness is brought into the Emergency Department. You diagnose it to be acute pulmonary edema. The patient does not respond to the standard treatment and is deteriorating rapidly in front of you. You know that the only treatment left is intubation and mechanical ventilation. As the patient is old and has multiple medical problems, including ischaemic heart disease and a left-sided stroke that left her semi-ambulant, and multiple admissions for acute pulmonary edema, you proceed to speak to her relatives first.

(a) Should you withhold intubation if the relatives tell you not to actively resuscitate the patient although the patient does not have a "Do not resuscitate" (DNR) order?

(b) If you withhold intubation and the patient dies, can her next of kin sue you?

(c) In a different scenario, you feel that a patient with terminal lung cancer who comes in hypotensive and tachypnoeic should not be intubated, but the relatives insist on active resuscitation. Should you follow the wishes of the relatives?

Answers

(a) Should you withhold intubation if the relatives tell you not to actively resuscitate the patient although the patient does not have a "Do not resuscitate" (DNR) order?

If the patient has a living will, then the procedures under the Advanced Medical Directives must be followed before withholding intubation. If the patient does not have a living will, then it is appropriate to speak to the patient's relatives under our culture. However, intubation cannot be withheld unless it can be justified as a medically futile case.

(b) If you withhold intubation and the patient dies, can her next of kin sue you?

No, the patient's next of kin cannot sue you, if it is a medically futile case. It is negligence only when it is not a "medically futile" case.

(c) In a different scenario, you feel that a patient with terminal lung cancer who comes in hypotensive and tachypnoeic should not be intubated, but the relatives insist on active resuscitation. Should you follow the wishes of the relatives?

You should try your best to explain to the patient's relatives about finite resources in healthcare and the need to be prudent in the use of healthcare resources. The final medical decision still lies with the doctor.

> **Take-home Message**
> Learn how to *implement* the Advanced Medical Directives correctly.

Case Scenario 10

Turning Away Patients – Concept of Vicarious Liability

A 28-year-old woman turns up at the Emergency Department complaining of fever and a rash of one-day duration. As it is a very busy shift with many patients still waiting to see the doctor, the triage nurse tells the patient that it will be better for her to consult a general practitioner (GP) instead. The woman goes home instead of seeing a GP that day. The following day, she is found to be comatosed and subsequently dies. The post-mortem examination reveals meningococcal meningitis as the cause of her death.

(a) Can the nurse be sued for turning the patient away?

(b) Can the hospital be sued?

(c) Is there any way of settling the family's claims instead of settlement through legal action?

Answers

(a) Can the nurse be sued for turning the patient away?

Yes, the nurse can be sued for not accepting patients in the Emergency Department. The nurse does not have the authority to turn away a patient. However, the following action will be acceptable: The nurse can inform the patient that the waiting time for consultation is long as there are many patients waiting to be seen. A list of possible alternative options to seek medical treatment is then given to the patient and the final decision is left to her.

(b) Can the hospital be sued?

The hospital can be sued for either vicarious liability for the actions of its nurse, or it can also be sued directly if there is no proper system (or protocol) for nurses to follow in such a situation, or the failure of such a system.

The nurse is an employee and agent of the hospital. The hospital is obliged to follow the *Bolam* test. If application of the test shows that the hospital should not have turned the patient away, then the hospital can be sued for negligence.

(c) Is there any way of settling the family's claims instead of settlement through legal action?

Yes. Many hospitals have an administrative department that has a legal officer or a person to deal with claims. Mediation or negotiation can be explored.

If the claim is not settled at this stage, lawyers may come into the picture and the hospital's lawyers should take over.

Take-home Message

There are various alternative dispute resolutions (ADRs) such as negotiations or consultations, mediation and arbitration to solve medical disputes.

HIV – Infectious Diseases Act;
When to Disclose Information

A 35-year-old married man comes to the Emergency Department complaining of a dry cough and weight loss of three weeks' duration, and shortness of breath for two days. On examination, the patient is noted to be febrile, very tachypnoeic and hypoxaemic, but the lung findings are relatively minimal. The chest x-ray done reveals diffuse interstitial infiltrates bilaterally. You suspect a diagnosis of pneumocystis carinii pneumonia.

(a) Do you need the patient's consent to test for Human Immuno-deficiency Virus (HIV) infection?

(b) If the HIV test turns out to be positive, does the treating doctor have a duty to
  (i) inform the patient's wife?
  (ii) report him to the health authorities under the Infectious Diseases Act?

Answers

(a) Do you need the patient's consent to test for Human Immuno-deficiency Virus (HIV) infection?

Ethically, yes, although there is no written law on this point. This is a case of "diagnostic testing" for the benefit of the patient. It is being done to enable the doctor to treat the patient for the ailments he has complained of. However, if it is done for other purposes such as to protect the doctors treating him, or for public benefit, consent should definitely be obtained.

(b) If the HIV test turns out to be positive, does the treating doctor have a duty to
(i) inform the patient's wife?

The treating doctor has a duty to inform his patient's wife only if he knows that the patient will not inform her. Under Section 25A of the Infectious Diseases Act (Cap. 137), a medical practitioner may disclose information relating to any person whom he reasonably believes to be infected with AIDS or HIV to the spouse, former spouse or any other contact of the infected person, or to a health officer for the purpose of making the disclosure to the spouse, former spouse or any other contact.

However, the medical practitioner cannot disclose any information unless

- he reasonably believes that it is medically appropriate, and that there is a significant risk of infection to the spouse, former spouse or any other contact;
- he has counselled the infected person on the need to notify the spouse, former spouse or any other contact, and he **reasonably believes that the infected person will not inform the spouse**, former spouse or other contact; and
- he has informed the infected person of his intent to make such disclosure to the spouse, former spouse or other contact.

Under Section 25(5) of the Infectious Diseases Act, if a medical practitioner is unable, by any reasonable means, to counsel or inform the infected person, he may apply to the Director of Medical Services to waive the above requirements. The Director may approve the application if, in the opinion of the Director, it is medically appropriate to disclose the information and that there is a significant risk of infection to the spouse, former spouse or other contact.

Further, no person can disclose such information to any person other than the infected person himself. Any person who disobeys will be guilty of an offence and shall be liable on conviction to a fine not exceeding $10,000 or to imprisonment for a term not exceeding three months or to both.

(ii) report him to the health authorities under the Infectious Diseases Act?

Yes, the treating doctor is bound by duty under the Infectious Diseases Act to notify the Director of Medical Services of any infectious diseases such as HIV. Under Section 6 of the Infectious Diseases Act, every medical practitioner who has reason to believe or suspect that any person attended to or treated by him is suffering from an infectious disease or is a carrier of that disease must notify the Director of Medical Services within the prescribed time and in such form or manner as the Director may require.

Under Section 6(2) of the Infectious Diseases Act, every person in charge of a laboratory used for the diagnosis of disease who becomes aware of the existence of an infectious disease in the course of his work must notify the Director within the prescribed time.

Under Section 6(5) of the Infectious Diseases Act, any person who fails to notify an infectious disease or furnishes as true information which he knows or has reason to believe to be false will be guilty of an offence. When such a person is charged for failing to report an infectious disease, he will be presumed to have known of the existence of the disease unless he proves to the satisfaction of the court that he had no such knowledge and could not with reasonable diligence have obtained such knowledge.

Every medical practitioner must report or notify the authorities of any of the infectious diseases specified in the First and Second Schedule of the Infectious Diseases Act.

First Schedule
Infectious Diseases
(1)   Acquired Immune Deficiency Syndrome
(1A)   Avian influenza
(2)   Chickenpox
(3)   Cholera
(4)   Dengue
(5)   Dengue haemorrhagic fever
(6)   Diphtheria

(7)   Encephalitis

(8)   Hand, foot and mouth disease

(9)   Human Immunodeficiency Virus Infection (Non-acquired Immune Deficiency Syndrome)

(10) Legionellosis

(11) Leprosy

(12) Malaria

(13) Measles

(14) Mumps

(15) Nipah virus infection

(16) Paratyphoid

(17) Plague

(18) Poliomyelitis

(19) Rubella

(20) Severe Acute Respiratory Syndrome (SARS)

(21) Typhoid

(22) Tuberculosis

(23) Venereal disease –

    (a) Chancroid   (d) Non-gonococcal urethritis

    (b) Genital herpes   (e) Syphilis

    (c) Gonorrhea

(24) Viral hepatitis

(25) Yellow fever

Second Schedule
Dangerous Infectious Diseases

(1)   Plague

(2)   Severe Acute Respiratory Syndrome (SARS)

(3)   Yellow fever

Take-home Message

Always check the First and Second Schedule, and any new updates on infectious diseases that need to be reported to the authorities. Ignorance of the law is no defence.

Allergic Reaction – Can Ignorance Be Used As Defence?

A patient is seen at the Emergency Department for a back sprain sustained after lifting some heavy objects. He tells the doctor that he is allergic to a medication but he does not know the name. The doctor gives him an intramuscular injection of diclofenac. The patient then develops periorbital edema, wheezing and hypotension. On tracing the patient's medical records subsequently, he is found to be allergic to diclofenac.

(a) Can the above doctor be sued if the patient dies from the allergic reaction?

(b) Does ignorance on the part of a patient absolve a doctor from blame should an untoward outcome result from the doctor's action?

Answers

(a) Can the above doctor be sued if the patient dies from the allergic reaction?

The doctor can be sued for negligence if the patient dies as a result of the intramuscular injection of diclofenac. Even if the patient does not die, the doctor is liable for negligence in not checking through the patient's medical records. Under the *Bolam* test (see Appendix 1 for further details), if another doctor in the same situation would have checked the patient's medical records for any history of allergies, then the above doctor should also have checked the medical records. As the above doctor did not check, he can be sued for negligence whether the patient dies or not.

Further, the patient should be advised to see a GP immediately if there is any allergic reaction, or to come back to the Emergency Department of the hospital immediately.

(b) Does ignorance on the part of a patient absolve a doctor from blame should an untoward outcome result from the doctor's action?

Even if a patient is unaware and ignorant of his allergies, the doctor can be deemed negligent if he does not check the patient's medical records for any allergies under the *Bolam* test.

If the patient has never been to that hospital, then the hospital will have no medical records of his allergies. The emergency doctor should still try his best to trace the patient's medical records as far as he can. This is especially so since medical records are kept in all public hospitals in Singapore and are accessible electronically nationwide.

Case Scenario 13

Intravenous Potassium Chloride Death – Gaps in Medical Knowledge; Censure

A newly graduated house officer gives an intravenous potassium chloride bolus to a patient leading to the patient's death. In his defence, the doctor claims that he was not taught that potassium cannot be given as a bolus in his medical school.

(a) Can a medical school be sued for gaps of knowledge in its curriculum?

(b) Will causing the unintentional death of a patient necessarily lead to that doctor being struck off the medical register so that he can no longer practise clinical medicine?

Answers

(a) Can a medical school be sued for gaps of knowledge in its curriculum?

The medical school can be sued if it is reasonably foreseeable that this omission in an appropriate part of the curriculum can make doctors a potential danger to society. It ultimately depends on the nature and type of omission. Doctors are meant to cure and not to kill.

Further, every doctor must be acting under supervision upon graduation from medical school. Under the *Bolam* test (see Appendix 1 for further details), the same standard of medical care applies even if you are young or inexperienced. Therefore, a newly graduated house officer must display the same standard of alertness and medical care as any other doctor in the particular field of medicine.

(b) Will causing the unintentional death of a patient necessarily lead to that doctor being struck off the medical register so that he can no longer practise clinical medicine?

Doctors do not easily get struck off the register. It is the ultimate punishment under the Medical Registration Act.

There are other punishments such as

- censure
- fine
- suspension up to three years and not less than three months

"Gross negligence" (a flexible term) should be accompanied by a conscious disregard for the welfare of a patient. A censure, or a censure and supervision, is more likely, if gross negligence leading to professional misconduct can be established.

Case Scenario 14

Informal Medical Consultation – Legal Implications

Doctor A is consulted by a friend informally over the phone about the condition of her four-year-old son who has fallen from a double-decker bed and hit the back of his head. There is no loss of consciousness or vomiting, but the friend is worried about a 4-cm bump at the back of his head. However, as it is bedtime, her son is asleep. Doctor A advises her friend that should her son be unarousable or develop vomiting, it will be best to bring him to the Emergency Department.

The following morning, the boy is found to be in a coma.

(a) Can a doctor be sued for an informal consultation?

(b) Can a doctor be liable should the medications prescribed for a friend without a formal consultation result in adverse consequences?

(c) What are the legal implications of a telephone consultation
   (i) between a caller and a healthcare worker working in the Emergency Department?

   (ii) between an emergency doctor and another doctor from another specialty who is on call and has not come down personally to examine the patient discussed?

Answers

(a) Can a doctor be sued for an informal consultation?

Yes, a doctor can be sued for negligent advice given during an informal consultation. See also the SMC Ethical Code with regard to remote initial consultations.

(b) Can a doctor be liable should the medications prescribed for a friend without a formal consultation result in adverse consequences?

Yes. A doctor can be liable whether it is a formal or informal consultation should adverse consequences occur due to the doctor's negligence.

Medications should not be prescribed over the phone or by fax or e-mail. See SMC Ethical Code 4.1.1.1 for the segment on adequate clinical evaluation.

(c) What are the legal implications of a telephone consultation
(i) between a caller and a healthcare worker working in the Emergency Department?

The medico-legal implications are the same whether it is a telephone consultation or a face-to-face consultation, although in a telephone consultation, the doctor will be giving medical advice based on the limited facts disclosed by the patient over the phone.

A healthcare worker such as a nurse is not entitled to give any medical advice to anybody whether on the phone or in person. However, if no damage has occurred, he or she cannot be successfully sued for negligence.

If there is breach of established protocol or guidelines, disciplinary action can be taken against that worker by the hospital. Further, the hospital is vicariously liable for the acts and omissions of all the healthcare workers in its employ.

(ii) between an emergency doctor and another doctor from another specialty who is on call and has not come down personally to examine the patient discussed?

As it is the duty of the doctor from another specialty who is on call to come down personally to examine the patient at the Emergency Department, he can be liable for negligence under the *Bolam* test if he does not see the patient. Hence the doctor on call will be liable for the telephone consultation.

The doctor on call may also be in breach of the SMC Ethical Code, and SMC may take disciplinary action against him. The hospital can also take its own disciplinary action against the doctor on call. A civil suit against him may be unsuccessful if he has not **caused** any damage.

Case Scenario 15

Death from Negligence;
Legal Implications of a Locum

Doctor B, a locum in the Emergency Department of hospital X, sees a 60-year-old man who complains of a headache of one-day duration. The onset of headache is not sudden but the patient has some associated giddiness. The patient says he is on some medications but he is unable to give their names. An examination of the patient does not reveal any neurological deficit. Doctor B gives the patient an injection of analgesics and his headache subsides. Doctor B diagnoses it as a tension headache and hence discharges the patient.

The following morning, the patient is found in a coma and brought to the Emergency Department again by his relatives. Among the patient's medications brought by the relatives is an anticoagulant, warfarin. An urgent CT scan taken shows an intracerebral haemorrhage. Unfortunately, an operation done thereafter could not save the patient and he dies two days later.

(a) Was Doctor B negligent as he did not know that the patient he saw was taking an anticoagulant and hence sent him home, and the patient subsequently went into a coma and died?

(b) Is Hospital X liable to be sued as well since Doctor B is only a locum and not one of its employees?

Answers

(a) Was Doctor B negligent as he did not know that the patient he saw was taking an anticoagulant and hence sent him home, and the patient subsequently went into a coma and died?

To determine whether Doctor B is negligent or not, apply the *Bolam* test (see Appendix 1) as supplemented by the *Bolitho* case (see Appendix 2). Should another emergency doctor have made further inquiries to find out if the patient is on anticoagulant medication, then Doctor B is negligent under the *Bolam* test. Therefore, it is important that Doctor B does what is the current accepted practice under the *Bolam* test. But the accepted current practice must withstand logical analysis such as those supported by evidence-based medicine.

Therefore, the question is whether the patient should have been sent home. If Doctor B had known that the patient was taking warfarin, the accepted practice is that he should not have sent the patient home without performing a CT brain scan first. Hence, Doctor B would be deemed negligent.

(b) Is Hospital X liable to be sued as well since Doctor B is only a locum and not one of its employees?

A locum at a hospital is generally considered an "independent contractor" and not an employee merely because he is "employed" by the hospital.

However, as locums are "agents" of the hospital in any case, the hospital is still vicariously liable. So Hospital X can be vicariously liable or responsible for all the wrongdoings and negligence of its employees and agents who act within the scope of their employment, including the locum Doctor B.

Pre-hospital Accidents – Legality to Check a Patient's Belongings; Reporting to the Authorities

A 40-year-old male who was involved in a high-speed traffic accident is brought by ambulance to the Emergency Department. He was riding home alone when he was thrown approximately 10 metres from his motorcycle after crashing into the road divider. He complains of shortness of breath and pain in his chest. He admits to drinking a "few beers" and taking some heroin prior to the accident. He has a carrier bag containing his personal documents.

(a) Is it legally acceptable to open the patient's carrier bag to access his personal documents given his condition?

(b) Must the nurse working in the Emergency Department report the patient's drug use to the authorities? How should such information given by a patient be documented?

Answers

(a) Is it legally acceptable to open the patient's carrier bag to access his personal documents given his condition?

If such documents will help the doctor in his medical treatment, then it is all right to look into the patient's carrier bag.

(b) Must the nurse working in the Emergency Department report the patient's drug use to the authorities? How should such information given by a patient be documented?

Yes, the nurse must report the patient's drug use of heroin before he met with the accident. The hospital should document in its notes that the patient had taken heroin.

Case Scenario 17

Research – Informed Consent

Your department is conducting research on a new procedure for treating scalp lacerations.

(a) What are all the essential steps involved in getting the consent of a patient who is being recruited for a research project?

(b) What happens if the patient to be recruited does not understand English and you do not speak the language that the patient understands?

Answers

(a) What are all the essential steps involved in getting the consent of a patient who is being recruited for a research project?

In clinical research trials, the research doctor must obtain informed consent from a research human subject who is the patient in this case. Informed consent is an ethical concept under the medical ethics of autonomy (self-respect or self-determination). The International Code of Ethics which includes the Declaration of Helsinki (Appendix 5), (US) Belmont Report (Appendix 6) and the International Conference on Harmonization (ICH) Guideline for Good Clinical Practice, stresses the importance of informed consent. The law of informed consent also makes the doctor liable for negligence if the patient has not given proper informed consent.

To ensure that clinical trials are conducted to internationally acceptable ethical and scientific standards, all investigators must comply with the Singapore Guideline for Good Clinical Practice (GCP) and the Medicines (Clinical Trials) Regulations. Paragraph 4.8 of the Singapore Guideline for GCP deals with "Informed Consent of Trial Subjects".

Before the trial starts, the investigator should have the written approval of the Ethics Committee (EC) or the Institutional Review Board (IRB) for the written informed consent form and any other written information to be given to the human subject. This written informed consent form or patient information sheet (PIS) should be revised whenever important new information becomes available that may be relevant to the subject's consent. Any revised written informed consent form and PIS should receive the EC's approval in advance of their use. The subject should be informed in a timely manner if new information becomes available that is relevant to the subject's willingness to continue participating in the trial. Such communication of this new information should be documented.

The investigator or trial staff should not coerce or unduly influence a subject to participate or to continue in a trial. The written informed consent form or PIS cannot waive the subject's legal rights or release the investigator, the institution and the sponsor from their liability for negligence.

The language used in the oral and written PIS about the trial, including the written informed consent form, must be as non-technical as practicable and should be understandable to the subject. The best practice here is that the written informed consent form can be understood by a ten-year-old child.

Before informed consent may be obtained, the investigator should give the subject ample time and opportunity to

- inquire about details of the trial
- decide whether or not to participate in the trial

All questions about the trial from the patient should be satisfactorily answered.

Before the subject participates in the trial, the written informed consent form should be signed and personally dated by

- the subject
- the person who conducts the informed consent discussion

If the subject is unable to read, an impartial witness should be present during the entire informed consent discussion. After the written informed consent form and PIS have been read and explained to the subject, the witness must sign and personally date the consent form. The witness should attest that

- the information in the consent form and PIS is accurately explained to, and apparently understood by, the subject
- informed consent is freely given by the subject

Both the informed consent discussion and the PIS must include the following 20 explanations:

(a) that the trial involves research

(b) the purpose of the trial

(c) the trial treatment(s) and the probability for random assignment to each treatment

(d) the trial procedures to be followed, including all invasive procedures

(e) the subject's responsibilities

(f) those aspects of the trial that are experimental

(g) the reasonably foreseeable risks or inconveniences to the subject and, when applicable, to an embryo, foetus or nursing infant

(h) the reasonably expected benefits. When there is no intended clinical benefit to the subject, the subject should be made aware of this.

(i) the alternative procedures(s) or course(s) of treatment that may be available to the subject, and their important potential benefits and risks

(j) the compensation and/or treatment available to the subject in the event of trial-related injury

(k) the anticipated pro-rated payment, if any, to the subject for participating in the trial

(l) the anticipated expenses, if any, to be incurred by the subject for participating in the trial

(m) that the subject's participation in the trial is voluntary, and that the subject may refuse to continue in the trial or withdraw from it, at any time, without any penalty or loss of benefits to which the subject is otherwise entitled

(n) that the monitor(s), the auditor(s), the Medical Clinical Research Committee (MCRC) and EC, and the Ministry of Health will be given direct access to the subject's original medical records for the verification of clinical trial procedures and/or data, without violating the confidentiality of the subject, to the extent allowed by the law and regulations; and that by signing a written informed consent form, the subject is authorizing such access

(o) that records identifying the subject will be kept confidential and, to the extent permitted by the law and regulations, will not be made publicly available. If the results of the trial are published, the subject's identity will remain confidential

(p) that the subject will be informed in a timely manner if information becomes available that may be relevant to the subject's willingness to continue participating in the trial

(q) the person(s) to contact
   • for further information regarding the trial and the rights of trial subjects, and
   • in the event of trial-related injury

(r) the foreseeable circumstances and/or reasons under which the subject's participation in the trial may be terminated

(s) the expected duration of the subject's participation in the trial

(t) the approximate number of subjects involved in the trial

Before the subject begins participation in the trial, the subject should receive a copy of the signed and dated written informed consent form and PIS. Further, during a subject's participation in the trial, the subject should receive a copy of the signed and dated consent form **updates** and a copy of any **amendments** to the PIS.

In emergency situations, when prior consent of the subject is not possible, the consent of the subject's legally acceptable representative should be taken. When prior consent of the subject is not possible and the subject's legally acceptable representative is not available, enrolment of the subject must be done in accordance with the measures described in the protocol, with documented approval by the MCRC and EC. This is to

- protect the rights, safety and well-being of the subject, and
- ensure compliance with the laws and regulations

Such regulatory requirements include **written certification** from the **principal investigator** and **two specialists** who are not involved in the trial that

(a) the person is facing a life-threatening situation which necessitates intervention

(b) the person is unable to give his consent as a result of his medical condition

(c) it is not feasible to request the consent of the person or to contact his legal representative within the crucial period in which treatment must be administered

(d) neither the person nor his legal representative nor any members of the person's family has informed the principal investigator of his objection to the person's participation in the clinical trial

The subject or his legally acceptable representative must be informed about the trial as soon as possible and the consent to continue should be requested.

When a clinical trial (therapeutic or non-therapeutic) includes subjects who can only be enrolled in the trial with the consent of the subject's legally acceptable representative (e.g. minors or patients with severe dementia), the subject should be informed about the trial to the extent compatible with the subject's understanding, and the subject should sign and personally date the written informed consent, if capable.

However, non-therapeutic trials may be conducted on subjects **with the consent** of a legally acceptable representative provided the following conditions are satisfied:

- the objectives of the trial cannot be met by means of a trial on subjects who can give their informed consent personally
- the foreseeable risks to the subjects are low
- the negative impact on the subject's well-being is minimized and low
- the trial is not prohibited by law
- the approval of the MCRC and the EC is expressly sought on the inclusion of such subjects, and with the written approval covering this aspect

Such trials, unless an exception is justified, should be conducted on patients with a disease or condition for which the investigational product is intended. The subjects in these trials should be closely monitored and withdrawn if they appear to be unduly distressed.

> **Take-home Message**
>
> In research ethics, always observe "beneficence" which means "do good". Therefore, in clinical trials, always reduce or minimize the risks and increase the benefits.

(b) What happens if the patient to be recruited does not understand English and you do not speak the language that the patient understands?

An official interpreter is needed during the informed consent discussion. In addition, an official translation of the informed consent documentation must be approved by the IRB/Ethics Committee. If not, the patient cannot be recruited into the study.

Falsification of Medical Records
v Good Documentation

A patient returns for a repeat visit at the Emergency Department. He claims that his diarrhoea and vomiting have persisted despite the treatment given at the Emergency Department. He also angrily accuses the previous doctor of being unprofessional as he had only examined him cursorily the day before.

(a) What are the issues involved in this case?

(b) When you proceed to investigate the case by looking through the past records, you find the medical records complete, in fact, over-complete. What do you think could have possibly happened?

CONTINUED

Answers

(a) What are the issues involved in this case?

Medical negligence may occur in three areas:

- misdiagnosis
- wrong treatment
- failure to obtain a valid proper informed consent

Proper history taking and clinical evaluation by an emergency doctor are critical to a proper and accurate diagnosis. Whether the above doctor is negligent or not in his diagnosis or medical treatment will depend on whether what he did is or is not a current accepted practice under the *Bolam* test (see Appendix 1).

It is important that a doctor properly documents a patient's first visit in his notes. The reason for this is evident in the case above when the patient at a repeat visit alleges that the doctor had only examined him cursorily the day before. The good documentation of a doctor's notes is very important, as anything that is not written down can be construed to mean that it did not happen. It is also a question of "proof" after all.

Take-home Message

Good notes = good defence
Bad notes = bad defence
No notes = no defence

The medico-legal issues involved in a patient's repeat visit include whether or not the doctor is negligent in his clinical and physical examination of the patient and whether the doctor has obtained the proper informed consent of his patient by advising him that should his symptoms persist, he should return to the Emergency Department. The doctor should therefore give full disclosure and information to his patient on what may happen when the patient goes home after his first visit at the Emergency Department. This highlights the importance of proper communication with a patient. Learn how to communicate with care to a patient to avoid any lawsuit.

> **Take-home Message**
> Practise good documentation.
> Practise good communication.

(b) When you proceed to investigate the case by looking through the past records, you find the medical records complete, in fact, over-complete. What do you think could have possibly happened?

If it is a template-based medical record where a doctor needs only to click on the various fields, an investigation should be conducted to determine if the doctor had filled in the medical records without examining some of the points typed in the medical records. This should be checked against what the patient says in his complaint to the Emergency Department. If the doctor had falsified medical records, his conduct will amount to professional misconduct and he can be dealt with by the Singapore Medical Council.

Defensive Medicine – How to Reduce the Risk of Being Sued

You are a junior medical officer. You have heard so much from your seniors about past medical lawsuits. You wonder whether you should practise "defensive medicine". If not, are there any other ways to reduce the risk of being sued?

Answers

"Defensive medicine" refers to medical practice that is directed at protecting a doctor from being sued rather than the care of a patient. In particular, it infers excessive and unnecessary investigations. Good lawyers reassure us that as long as we practise safe and preferably evidence-based medicine, we cannot be successfully sued and that "defensive medicine" is unnecessary. In fact, practising defensive medicine may lead to a doctor being sued under the *Bolam* test (see Appendix 1) because it is not the current accepted practice to order unnecessary tests. The *Bolam* test is a defence for doctors, but it can also be used as a weapon by patients to sue doctors.

It is best to practise defensive documentation and good communication with patients.

Here are some tips to avoid being sued.

1. Build good rapport

One of the best ways to avert either a complaint or worse still, a lawsuit, is to build good rapport with patients and their relatives. Even if a genuine mistake occurs, patients and their relatives are more likely to excuse you if you have built good rapport with them. Suing is often one way of getting even with the arrogant and condescending healthcare professional. Should an error occur, it is often advisable to show absolute openness and frankness. This does not require an admission of negligence. Evasiveness will arouse the curiosity of the patient and his family, and make them go to great lengths to uncover the error. Always make liberal use of informed consent should you conduct any procedures that carry some risk.

2. Keep good documentation

Good notes will always be your best defence. It may just be one of the thousands of the emergency doctor's medical records, but it is most likely to be the only one for the patient. Hence, unless you document properly, the judge is more likely to believe what the patient says rather than what you say if it is not in the medical records. Slipshod notes are likely to indicate a slipshod doctor as well.

If you need to make subsequent additional notes, make sure they are properly dated and identified as such. Alteration of existing notes will be recognized as dishonest.

3. Refer to other doctors appropriately

Know your limitations and refer to or consult your seniors. Just remember that asking the opinion of your peers or juniors may not legally cover you.

4. Do not belittle a patient's complaints

A patient's complaints may at first glance appear to be trivial and not warrant an emergency consultation. However, just remember that a non-urgent diagnosis should always be a diagnosis by exclusion. Never turn a patient away from the Emergency Department without a proper assessment unless you wish to invite a complaint or lawsuit.

5. Make sure you have a valid medical practice insurance cover

It is prudent never to practise medicine unless you have a valid medical practice insurance cover as one can never know when a case may end up in a lawsuit.

6. Be aware of "red flags" situations:

- Change of shift.
- Patients returning to the Emergency Department for re-evaluation. Always review the previous medical charts of such patients.
- High risk medical encounters at the Emergency Department. Know what they are.
- Patients who frequently show up at the Emergency Department or are alcohol or drug abusers.

7. Follow hospital protocols

It is assumed that hospital protocols generally indicate the standard of care of that hospital. Hence, therapies that are aberrant from written hospital protocols are difficult to defend in court.

8. Do not over-rely on test results

Always remember that there is no perfect test in medicine. Know the limitations of the tests so that you can interpret them correctly.

9. Obtain old medical charts frequently

Make it a habit to always try to obtain the previous medical records of a patient as far as possible. This should help to increase the diagnostic accuracy of the patient as well as prevent medication errors.

Impending Lawsuit – When to Suspect It and How to Prepare for It

A patient whom you have treated recently keeps coming back to the Emergency Department to ask you for details about the management of his case. You are worried that this may be an ominous sign of a looming lawsuit.

(a) What are some of the signs of an impending lawsuit?

(b) What should you do if you suspect an impending lawsuit?

(c) Can presentations made during the department's morbidity and mortality round be used as evidence against the doctor in court?

(d) Is there a danger of the reporting of an adverse outcome or medical error in the hospital's occurrence reporting system being used against the doctor in court?

(e) How should a doctor prepare for legal action against himself?

(f) What does a doctor need to do to prepare himself as a professional witness in court?

(g) What is the difference between writing an ordinary medical report as opposed to an expert medical report?

CONTINUED ON

Answers

(a) What are some of the signs of an impending lawsuit?
- Patient calls frequently.
- Patient brings family or "friend" to see you.
- Patient asks very specific questions and writes down or tapes answers.
- Patient asks for a second opinion, after the procedure is done.
- Patient asks for medical records.
- Patient writes to you or your hospital, asking questions or for an explanation.
- Patient's lawyer writes to you.

(b) What should you do if you suspect an impending lawsuit?

You should notify your superior, staff and defence organization. Record down all conversations and correspondence. Organize your thoughts and recollections of the case. Organize the patient's medical records. Review to check if what you did is correct. Review as to who should be your expert witness.

In the meantime, all the patient's questions should be answered satisfactorily and promptly without delay. Do not be defensive or arrogant. Do not hope the matter will go away by itself. Deal with every question raised by the patient. Do not embellish or reconstruct. Do not hide or destroy evidence.

(c) Can presentations made during the department's morbidity and mortality round be used as evidence against the doctor in court?

Yes. The process of discovery will require all medical records and presentations made during the department's morbidity and mortality round to be given to the patient and his lawyers in a lawsuit.

(d) Is there a danger of the reporting of an adverse outcome or medical error in the hospital's occurrence reporting system being used against the doctor in court?

In the case of *Riverside Hosp. v Johnson* (2006), the Virginia Supreme Court held that incident reports presented to the hospital's quality control committee were not privileged under the states' peer review statutes because they were factual information collected in the ordinary course of business and operations of the hospital.

The contributing editor, Robert A Bitterman, in the *ED Legal Letter*, June 2007, Vol. 17, No. 6, wrote:

> Many health care providers harbor the delusion that hospital "incident reports" or "occurrence screens," are privileged and protected from discovery or admission as evidence against them in malpractice litigation. A rash of recent court decisions dispels that notion …

However, any notes or reports for audit purposes cannot be discovered by the patient and his lawyers in the process of discovery in a lawsuit.

(e) How should a doctor prepare for legal action against himself?

Usually, legal action is first threatened through a letter written by the patient or a "demand letter" from a lawyer outlining the negligence involved and a demand for extravagant compensation.

The doctor is to inform the protection organization covering him or his insurance company. In fact, they have to be alerted as soon as the adverse outcome has taken place, and common sense dictates that there could be a future possible claim. The demands for compensation come later.

The doctor is then to see the lawyer he has chosen or who has been recommended to him, to explain in detail the facts involved, which is to be accompanied by a written report labelled as the "First Incident Report". At this stage, what is told or written by the doctor is bound to be incomplete. The doctor must keep trying to recall what other facts exist, work out whether the case is defensible or indefensible and inform his lawyer of the areas where he could be vulnerable or blameworthy.

Depending on the stage of the threatened legal action, there will be more interaction between the doctor and the lawyers. For example, the reply to the demand letter will have to be carefully crafted; the doctor must give proper input and check carefully whatever his lawyers write to the other party. Further, this will be the time to identify an expert witness and to get his report.

With effect from 1 January 2007, the Pre-action Protocol for Medical Negligence Claims issued by the Subordinate Courts applies to all cases not exceeding $250,000. Under the said protocol, medical reports have to be given, and explanations must be given by the doctor to the patient face to face. At such meetings, lawyers will also be present so that not only liability but the total package of general damages, special damages, loss of earnings (if any) and future medical expenses (if any) can be thrashed out. The doctor must therefore be prepared to explain convincingly to the patient (with diagrams or pictures, if possible) what had happened and that he has tried his best. If matters are settled at this stage, the matter ends.

If the matter does not end here, the patient will start legal proceedings through his lawyer by filing a writ and statement of claim. The doctor will again be required to see his lawyer to give more facts and his views to counter the allegations in the statement of claim. After a defence is filed on behalf of the doctor, there will be a reply on behalf of the doctor and pleadings will be closed. Thereafter the matter will go for a possible settlement before a "settlement judge" in the Court Dispute Resolution Centre of the Subordinate Courts.

The doctor will be required to assist his lawyer in preparing a summary of events for the settlement judge and submit all necessary documents prior to the settlement sessions. The lawyers will then proceed with such settlement proceedings and the doctor's presence will thereafter not be necessary. However, as there may be one or more sessions before the settlement judge, the doctor must assist his lawyer by giving further facts or documents (if any) to counter any allegations put forward by the other party for the next settlement session. Usually, things are settled at this stage.

If matters are still not settled, and there is the possibility of a full blown trial, the doctor will have to assist his lawyer in preparing his affidavit of evidence-in-chief (AEIC), which is a detailed document in lieu of leading evidence-in-chief at the trial. The doctor will also have to assist his lawyer in getting an AEIC from his expert witness, or supplementary expert reports, as more issues will have surfaced from the time the statement of claim is filed for the patient.

If the trial proceeds, the doctor will have to go through all the documents and events that have taken place in the legal proceedings, and prepare for a prolonged and stressful cross-examination by the patient's lawyer.

At the end of the trial, there may be written submissions requiring the doctor's input; he must also give his views on what his own witnesses (not experts) have said, with regard to what the patient's witnesses (and experts) have said.

All in all, the doctor may be involved at many stages from the time legal action is threatened by the patient.

(f) What does a doctor need to do to prepare himself as a professional witness in court?

Here, the doctor is not a defendant in the suit, but may be a witness for the patient (plaintiff) or the defence. He is also not being called as an expert witness, but as a witness of fact. He may have treated the patient, or be able to assist the defence as a witness of fact, e.g. he could have dealt with a similar case, or he may have been involved at a later stage, either as a physician or surgeon to the patient.

In such cases, the doctor will be interviewed by the lawyer for whom he is called as a witness. A report or statement will be expected of him even before the writ or statement of claim is filed. Alternatively, it may be used at the settlement stage before the settlement judge of the Court Dispute Resolution Centre of the Subordinate Courts.

If the matter goes further, the doctor may be asked to give a more detailed affidavit of evidence-in-chief which will be sworn before a commissioner for oaths for use at the trial.

If the trial really goes on (things can be settled at any time), the doctor will normally have to see the lawyer concerned to go through all the relevant facts again so that he will be prepared for cross-examination by the lawyer for the opposite side.

(g) What is the difference between an ordinary medical report as opposed to an expert medical report?

An ordinary medical report will be either a report from the treating doctors or a report from a specialist who has seen or examined the patient, which will then be labelled as a "specialist report".

An expert medical report, on the other hand, is one that is not given by the treating doctors or doctors who are witnesses of fact. It involves an expert opinion from a senior doctor who is a specialist in his field, whose opinions will be considered by the court in legal proceedings, under Section 47 of the Evidence Act.

Expert reports, which may be obtained in anticipation of legal proceedings, should be given only after proper instructions from the doctor's lawyer to the expert. The expert should concentrate on the issues raised by the lawyer and enclose all relevant documents with his report.

Occasionally, expert reports may be obtained only after legal proceedings have been instituted. Aside from all other documents, the statement of claim and defence should be enclosed for his perusal. The expert can then dwell on the issues that have been raised or highlighted by the lawyer, and any other areas that he may deem necessary to include in his report.

Where expert reports have been given prior to legal proceedings, the expert can submit a further or supplementary report, dealing with the issues raised in the pleadings, which he has not seen before.

Case Scenario 21

Jehovah's Witness – Dilemma of Refusal of Blood Transfusion

A patient who is a Jehovah's Witness (JW) is brought to the Emergency Department by ambulance. He is in hypovolaemic shock following a road accident.

(a) If the patient is a competent adult who refuses to be given a blood transfusion, what should you do as the treating physician?

(b) If the patient is drowsy and his relatives claim that he is a JW, and therefore should not be given a blood transfusion, what should you do as the treating physician?

(c) What should you do as the treating physician if the patient is a child and his parents refuse to let him have a blood transfusion as he is a JW?

Answers

(a) If the patient is a competent adult who refuses to be given a blood transfusion, what should you do as the treating physician?

Assuming the patient is competent, the patient's wishes must be respected, whether or not this is due to him being a JW or belonging to some other system of belief or religion. A doctor cannot give a patient a blood transfusion without the patient's consent. The doctor should record in his notes the fact that the doctor has informed the patient of the full risks and implications of not giving him a blood transfusion and also, the fact of the patient's express refusal to receive the blood transfusion, notwithstanding what he has been told.

If, however, the doctor suspects for any good reason that the patient is incompetent to decide whether he should receive treatment or not (e.g. the patient is delirious or under the influence of some psychosis – for instance, he believes that he is a superhero and has magical healing powers), then the doctor has to act in the patient's best interests. This may include giving the patient a blood transfusion if that is warranted.

(b) If the patient is drowsy and his relatives claim that he is a JW, and therefore should not be given a blood transfusion, what should you do as the treating physician?

As in the answer to (a) above, the doctor must act in the patient's best interests since the patient is incompetent. The doctor can have regard to what the patient's relatives tell him as a guide as to what the patient would say if he could express his wishes, but that is where the reliance on the relatives' wishes ends. The doctor is not obliged to follow the instructions of the patient's relatives blindly.

As such, if the doctor feels that he must err on the side of caution in acting in the patient's best interests, and a blood transfusion is indicated, the doctor should proceed with the transfusion.

This entire process should be clearly documented in the doctor's notes.

(c) **What should you do as the treating physician if the patient is a child and his parents refuse to let him have a blood transfusion as he is a JW?**

The parents, not the doctor, are the lawful guardians of the child. They exercise the child's autonomy for him. As such, if the parents of a child refuse to allow him to have a blood transfusion on the grounds that he is a JW, the doctor must respect those wishes, clearly documenting that he has been refused consent to proceed with the blood transfusion.

If the blood transfusion is a treatment that is absolutely necessary to save the child's life, the doctor may also wish to warn the parents of the child that they may be committing an offence under section 299 or 300 of the Penal Code which deals with culpable homicide and murder. Section 299 reads:

> **299.** Whoever causes death by doing an act with the intention of causing death, or with the intention of causing such bodily injury as is likely to cause death, **or with the knowledge that he is likely by such act to cause death,** commits the offence of culpable homicide.

The Penal Code says that an "act" includes "an illegal omission" – Section 32.

In this case, the illegal omission is the parents' refusal to give consent for their child to receive the blood transfusion.

As a matter of prudence, the doctor should also report the parents' refusal to the police and note down all that he has told the parents, and their response, in detail, in his notes.

Case Scenario 22

Plane Doctor – Medical Ethics on "Not Helping"

You are on board a plane. A passenger becomes breathless and collapses. Diagnosing a tension pneumothorax on one side, you attempt to treat him with a sharp object. Unfortunately, the patient dies from bleeding from a punctured lung.

(a) If you have not come forward to help and it is discovered later that you are a doctor, can you be sued?

(b) Can the person's relatives sue you for causing harm should your treatment cause some adverse outcome instead?

CONTINUED ON

Answers

(a) If you have not come forward to help and it is discovered later that you are a doctor, can you be sued?

Under medical ethics, a doctor should come forward to help the passenger. Legally, you are under no duty to come to the rescue of a passer-by.

(b) Can the person's relatives sue you for causing harm should your treatment cause some adverse outcome instead?

Under such circumstances, a doctor is not liable as he is treating the person with limited resources outside a hospital setting. However, should a doctor be found to be wantonly negligent, he can be sued for negligence.

Take-home Message

In medical ethics of beneficence, every doctor should come forward to help in a situation where his professional expertise is needed.

Case Scenario 23

Voluntary Medical Practitioner – Bound by the Same Rules?

A doctor running a clinic on a voluntary basis prescribes a medication that leads to a fatal drug allergic reaction in his patient.

Is a voluntary medical practitioner legally bound by the same rules as a regular doctor who receives a fee for his services?

Answers

Is a voluntary medical practitioner bound by the same rules legally as a regular doctor who receives fees for service?

Yes. A voluntary doctor is legally bound by the same laws even if he gives free medical treatment; he is still liable for negligence in the same way as a regular doctor who charges medical consultation fees.

Take-home Message

You are still liable for negligence even if you provide free medical consultations or services.

Case Scenario 24

Human Organ Transplant Act (HOTA)

A patient who was involved in a road accident suffers brain death. His family members are not willing to let his organs be removed under the Human Organ Transplant Act (HOTA).

(a) What is HOTA?

(b) Does HOTA apply to all citizens, permanent residents and even non-citizens?

(c) How are Muslims affected under HOTA?

(d) Can family members refuse to let the organs be removed from a brain-dead patient if the patient had not opted out of HOTA?

CONTINUED ON

Answers

(a) What is HOTA?

The Human Organ Transplant Act (HOTA) covers all non-Muslim Singapore citizens and permanent residents between the ages of 21 and 60. Muslims are not covered for religious reasons. (At the time of writing this book, there have been discussions for HOTA to apply to Muslims as well.) HOTA does not apply to persons of unsound mind unless the parent or guardian consents. HOTA does not apply to foreigners. However, they can still use the Medical (Therapy, Education and Research) Act (METRA) to donate their organs for research as anatomical gifts.

HOTA confers priority in receiving a cadaveric organ, where required. Hence, those who opt out of HOTA (including persons not covered by HOTA) will receive lower priority on the organ transplant wait list. People can opt out of HOTA if they do not wish to donate their organs when they die. They must mention the specific organ they do not want to donate.

Since 1 July 2004, HOTA covers

- the liver, heart and cornea, in addition to the kidney, in the case of a donor's death
- both accidental and non-accidental deaths
- living donor organ transplantation

However, HOTA does not have any provisions whereby one can specify the organ recipient or specifically exclude persons from being organ recipients. HOTA does not govern the removal or the use of organs removed incidental to a surgical procedure on a living person who has consented to the organ removal or in a life-saving situation.

Living donor organ transplantation is prohibited except in certain situations where the following criteria must be met:

- Written authorization must be obtained from the Transplant Ethics Committee (TEC).
- TEC must be satisfied that the donor thoroughly understands the nature and consequences of the medical procedures.
- TEC must be satisfied that the donor has given his full informed consent.
- TEC must be satisfied that there is no emotional coercion or financial inducement involved in the donor's decision to donate the organ.

Contracts for trade in organs or blood are void. Anyone who trades in organs or blood can be fined up to $10,000 and/or jailed for up to one year. The advertising of the sale of organs or blood is prohibited under HOTA.

(b) Does HOTA apply to all citizens, permanent residents and even non-citizens?

HOTA applies only to Singapore citizens and Singapore permanent residents. It does not apply to foreigners.

(c) How are Muslims affected under HOTA?

Muslims are not governed by HOTA. They will receive lower priority on the organ transplant wait list. (However, at the time of writing this book, there have been discussions for HOTA to apply to Muslims as well.)

(d) Can family members refuse to let the organs be removed from a brain-dead patient if the patient had not opted out of HOTA?

The family members cannot refuse.

Refusal of a Doctor to Attend to a Pre-hospital Patient

A motorcyclist skids and is flung off his motorcycle. He lands just in front of a general practitioner's (GP) clinic. A passer-by goes to the GP to ask him to attend to the injured motorcyclist. The GP refuses, saying that he cannot do much. Instead, he will just call for an ambulance to bring the accident victim to the Emergency Department. The patient dies by the time the ambulance arrives.

(a) Can the GP be sued for refusing to attend to an injured person who is not one of his patients?

(b) Can the GP give the excuse that he is not proficient enough to handle a certain clinical condition because of inadequate expertise or equipment?

Answers

(a) Can the GP be sued for refusing to attend to an injured person who is not one of his patients?

The GP has no legal duty to come to the rescue of that injured person. He is, however, bound by medical ethics to assist an injured person. (See SMC Ethical Code and Guidelines.) In this case, the GP can be subject to professional disciplinary proceedings by the Singapore Medical Council.

(b) Can the GP give the excuse that he is not proficient enough to handle a certain clinical condition because of inadequate expertise or equipment?

The GP should ethically still try his best to assist the injured motorcyclist with his limited resources. He can at least administer first aid or basic trauma life support procedures.

It is fundamental that a doctor should not do what he cannot do, but he must assist as much as possible, such as calling an ambulance immediately and going with the injured person in the ambulance to the hospital.

Take-home Message

Under medical ethics, doctors must help strangers in distress, even when they are not their patients.

Case Scenario 26

Illegal Prescription of Controlled Drugs – Legal Implications

A GP is found to have prescribed controlled drugs for a patient who has no real indication of needing it.

(a) What is the penalty for a doctor found to be prescribing controlled drugs illegally?

(b) Does the doctor run the risk of being struck off the medical register for such conduct?

Answers

(a) What is the penalty for a doctor found to be prescribing controlled drugs illegally?

The doctor can be fined or suspended by the Singapore Medical Council for professional misconduct in endangering the life of a patient.

(b) Does the doctor run the risk of being struck off the medical register for such conduct?

Yes, the doctor can be struck off the medical register.

Take-home Message

Always act in the best interests of patients for their safety and well-being.
Know the law and regulations.
Comply with them!

Case Scenario 27

False Accusation Against a Doctor

A male GP is accused by a female patient of molesting her. He had examined her chest without a chaperone.

(a) How should this complaint be handled?

(b) If the accusation turns out to be true, what is the likely penalty for the GP?

(c) What are some of the ways to prevent false accusations by a patient?

Answers

(a) How should this complaint be handled?

In many cases, the complaint is not reported to the police if it involves only an examination with no molestation. The complaint may be made to the SMA or SMC. It is wise to consult a lawyer immediately in all cases of complaint, whenever one is made.

(b) If the accusation turns out to be true, what is the likely penalty for the GP?

The mere absence of a chaperone may not even be regarded as professional misconduct, depending on the explanations given by the doctor to the SMC. There have been cases where the Complaints Committee of the SMC has only given written advice or warning to the doctor as allowed under the Medical Registration Act.

(c) What are some of the ways to prevent false accusations by a patient?

Having a chaperone is one way. The other way is to tell the patient that a chaperone is not available and get the patient's express consent for an examination. Another alternative is to ask her to bring into the consultation room her friend or relative who may have come with her.

> **Take-home Message**
> Always have someone around during clinical examination.

Patient's Verbal Abuse of Doctor — What Legal Recourse Does the Doctor Have?

A patient shouts abusive language at a doctor and also threatens to harm her. The patient soon starts stalking the doctor wherever she goes.

(a) Can the doctor seek any legal redress?

(b) What can the doctor do to protect herself from harm?

Answers

(a) Can the doctor seek any legal redress?

There can be legal redress only if a tort, crime or breach of contract has been committed. As there is hardly any "damage", it will be foolhardy to sue in tort. Regarding a crime, see the Penal Code (Cap. 224) or the Miscellaneous Offences (Public Order and Nuisance) Act.

Firstly, there may be no crime at all, depending on the facts. There is also the legal principle of *de minimis lex* (i.e. the law will not consider trivial matters).

The abusive language is not an offence under the Penal Code, but may be an offence under the Miscellaneous Offences (Public Order and Nuisance) Act.

The threat to harm may amount to "criminal intimidation" under Section 503 of the Penal Code.

The "stalking" may amount to the criminal offence of harassment, alarm or distress under Section 13B of the Miscellaneous Offences (Public Order and Nuisance) Act.

However, it is important to ascertain the facts that made the patient abusive. Could there have been long delays or undue provocation on the part of the doctor such as arrogant behaviour?

(b) What can the doctor do to protect herself from harm?

Reporting to the police will not prevent harm. The police have to be called at the time when the patient threatens to harm the doctor. Even then, any harm that may be caused by the patient may have already befallen the doctor before the police arrive.

In the Singapore context, stalkers hardly exist. There may be rare cases where the doctor is a young and attractive female. She can consider employing a bodyguard to protect herself from stalkers.

The doctor can employ a big-sized man as a "bouncer" to eject the patient from the clinic, which is within the law. A cheap and effective remedy will be to meet "hate" with "love". Calm down the angry patient, apologize to him and show empathy. A diplomatic female clinic manager or a female clinic nurse or assistant can also help to defuse the situation.

Take-home Message

When emotions run high, stay calm.

Do not provoke the person or be arrogant.

Be helpful and caring.

Always ask ourselves: "Did we contribute to such a situation?"

Case Scenario 29

Research — Waiver of Informed Consent

You want to conduct a research to determine which drug (A or B) is more effective in successfully reviving a patient from cardiac arrest. However, you know that it will be impossible to get the consent of patients at the Emergency Department because they are usually in a collapsed state or a critically ill state.

(a) Is informed consent always required in the conduct of all types of clinical research? Are there any exceptions to the rule?

(b) Can or should the informed consent be obtained from the next of kin?

Answers

(a) Is informed consent always required in the conduct of all types of clinical research? Are there any exceptions to the rule?

The ethical concept of informed consent is crucial in any clinical research study. So informed consent must be obtained at all times, unless the five conditions listed below are satisfied. The Institutional Review Board (IRB) or Ethics Committee may approve a consent procedure that does not include, or which alters, some or all of the elements of informed consent, or waive the requirement to obtain informed consent provided the IRB finds and documents that

(i)   The research involves no more than minimal risk to the subjects.

(ii)   The waiver or alteration will not adversely affect the rights and welfare of the subjects.

(iii) Whenever appropriate, the subjects will be provided with additional pertinent information after participation.

(iv)   The research could not practicably be carried out without the waiver or alteration.

(v)   The research is not subject to FDA regulations.

A doctor or principal investigator cannot waive the requirement of informed consent. It is for the Ethics Committee or the IRB to waive informed consent under the above five conditions. A doctor or principal investigator cannot dispense with informed consent without the approval of the IRB.

Further, under the Singapore Guideline for Good Clinical Practice, paragraph 4.8.15, in emergency situations, where it is not possible to obtain the prior consent of the subject, the consent of the subject's legally acceptable representative, if present, should be requested.

When it is not possible to obtain the prior consent of the subject, and the subject's legally acceptable representative is not available, enrolment of the subject requires measures described in the protocol and/or elsewhere, with documented approval by the MCRC and Ethics Committee, or the IRB, to protect the rights, safety and well-being of the subject, and to ensure compliance with applicable regulatory requirements.

The latter regulatory requirements include written certification from the principal investigator and two other specialists who are not involved in the trial that

(i)   the person is facing a life-threatening situation which necessitates intervention

(ii) the person is unable to give his consent as a result of his medical condition

(iii) it is not feasible to request the consent of the person or to contact his legal representative within the crucial period in which treatment must be administered

(iv) neither the person nor his legal representative nor any members of the person's family has informed the principal investigator of his objection to the person's participation in the clinical trial

The subject or the subject's legally acceptable representative must be informed about the trial as soon as possible and the **consent to continue** and **any other consent** deemed appropriate **must be requested**.

(b) Can or should the informed consent be obtained from the next of kin?

No, consent cannot be obtained from the next of kin. See answer to (a) above.

Death from Aspiration — "Foreseeable" Harm

A 35-year-old man arrives at the Emergency Department with a dislocated upper left arm after a motorcycle accident. The emergency doctor does an X-ray and gives the patient conscious sedation before reducing the dislocation by Kocher's method. The doctor then leaves the patient in bed in the supine position to recover. In the meantime, when the doctor is busy with another patient, the patient wakes up choking on his own vomitus due to nausea from the sedatives. The patient subsequently dies.

Can the patient's relatives sue the doctor for causing the death of the patient due to negligence?

Answers

Can the patient's relatives sue the doctor for causing the death of the patient due to negligence?

This is a medico-legal case as the emergency doctor could have reasonably foreseen that a patient could choke on his own vomitus if he did not log-roll the patient to lie on his side, rather than putting him in a supine position. To prove that the doctor is negligent, the patient's relatives have to prove the four elements of:

- duty of care owed to the patient
- breach of duty of care by the doctor (standard of care is the *Bolam* test as supplemented by the *Bolitho* case)
- **causation** (doctor caused the death)
- **foreseeability** (damage not too remote)

The main issue based on the given facts will be to determine if there is a breach of a reasonable standard of medical care (i.e. breach of duty under the *Bolam* test).

Take-home Message

Always **foresee** what can cause harm to a patient.

Anything within the doctor's control is a **causation** factor for an act of negligence.

Informed Consent of the
Mentally Subnormal Individual

A 45-year-old mentally subnormal female with commercially available cyanoacrylate plastering the right side of her face and causing her eyes to remain shut is brought to the Emergency Department by her mentally subnormal male partner who requests for assistance to remove the cyanoacrylate. The patient is highly resistant to its removal due to psychogenic fears of pain during its removal and is vocal in her resistance during the process of removal.

(a) Can a mentally subnormal individual give valid consent *not* to receive treatment? What constitutes valid non-consent?

(b) Is the consent of the mentally subnormal partner valid?

Answers

(a) Can a mentally subnormal individual give valid consent *not* to receive treatment? What constitutes valid non-consent?

Under the law for informed consent, you must obtain the patient's consent before you remove the cyanoacrylate. However, since the patient is mentally subnormal, valid consent can be given by a Committee of Persons appointed by the court. If there is no appointment of a Committee of Persons, then the doctor has to treat the patient in her best interests.

(b) Is the consent of the mentally subnormal partner valid?

No, because no person can give consent for another person. Even if the boyfriend were not mentally subnormal, he cannot give consent unless he is appointed to the Committee of Persons by the court.

> **Take-home Message**
>
> Be familiar with the ethics and the law of informed consent for mentally impaired persons.

Non-adherence to Duty of Care – Legal Recourse

A 54-year-old female patient arrives at the Emergency Department with symptoms of sinusitis, eye discomfort, restricted extraocular movements and fullness of the right orbit. The attending medical officer treats the patient for pre-septal cellulitis with the appropriate oral antibiotics.

The patient is referred to the ophthalmology outpatient clinic with an appointment for two days later. There, she is seen by the consultant on call and a CT scan reveals the presence of a subperiosteal abscess secondary to contiguous sinusitis. The patient is admitted for intravenous antibiotics.

(a) Are there grounds for the patient to pursue legal action in a situation where a duty of care has not been followed (in this instance, same day orbit CT scan and admission for IV antibiotics)?

(b) Will there be grounds for legal recourse in the situation where clinical recovery is potentially delayed by non-adherence to the duty of care? How is compensation determined in such an instance?

Answers

(a) Are there grounds for the patient to pursue legal action in a situation where a duty of care has not been followed (in this instance, same day orbit CT scan and admission for IV antibiotics)?

If what the attending emergency doctor did is accepted current practice, that is not to refer to an ophthalmologist in the given situation, then he will not be liable for negligence under the *Bolam* test. If it is accepted current practice in the given case to give a same day orbit CT scan and admission for IV antibiotics, then the attending doctor is negligent.

(b) Will there be grounds for legal recourse in the situation where clinical recovery is potentially delayed by non-adherence to the duty of care? How is compensation determined in such an instance?

Yes, the patient can sue for damages, if clinical recovery is delayed by a breach of the doctor's duty of care. The monetary compensation will include damages for

- pain and suffering
- medical expenses
- hospital fees
- actual loss of earnings
- future loss of earnings, if the injury is likely to incapacitate the patient
- loss of amenities such as the loss of job satisfaction and the loss of leisure activities

In *Tay Cheng Yan v Tock Hua Bin* (1990), the court awarded the patient $25,000 for pain and suffering due to an injury to the left eye, $10,000 for injury to the skull and $2,500 for the fracture of two teeth. In another case of *Heng Kim Eng v SBS Ltd* (1978), the patient was awarded $28,000 in damages for pain and suffering due to the loss of the right eye.

Take-home Message
Refer a patient to a consultant in a timely manner.

Case Scenario 33

Missed Diagnosis of Strabismus and Exotropia and Failure to Refer to Consultant Ophthalmologist – GP Practice

A three-year-old girl is brought to the general practitioner (GP) because her parents feel that her eyes are not straight and are worried that she may have a squint. After using a torchlight to look at the corneal reflexes (Hirschberg test), the GP assures them that she does not have strabismus. Four years later, her parents feel that her eyes are drifting out more; the child is seen by an ophthalmologist who diagnoses her as having exotropia with loss of depth perception. The girl has intermittent exotropia, which has now broken down into a manifest exotropia.

(a) The GP examined the girl's eyes for strabismus using the corneal light reflex test, which can only detect manifest strabismus. As he did not go on to examine her eyes using the cover/uncover test and the alternate cover test, he could not detect latent strabismus. He also examined her only for near and not far distance. Was he negligent?

(b) Intermittent exotropia starts out as a latent exophoria and surgical intervention is indicated when the frequency of breakdown to a manifest exotropia is significant. Even if the girl had been seen and diagnosed with it when she was three, she may not have needed surgery at that point in time. Does that make the GP not liable?

Answers

(a) The GP examined the girl's eyes for strabismus using the corneal light reflex test, which can only detect manifest strabismus. As he did not go on to examine her eyes using the cover/uncover test and the alternate cover test, he could not detect latent strabismus. He also examined her only for near and not far distance. Was he negligent?

The *Bolam* test applies. Did he do what any responsible and competent GP would have done? If so, does that practice stand up to logic? For instance, if any responsible and competent GP would have done what the above GP did, then the above GP was not negligent. However, if any responsible and competent GP would have told the child's parents about the limitations of his test, and that it could not exclude latent strabismus, which the above GP had failed to do, then the above GP's care was substandard on that count. He can be made liable for negligence, if the child's parents can prove that their child's latent strabismus could have been treated successfully if it had been detected at that point in time.

(b) Intermittent exotropia starts out as a latent exophoria and surgical intervention is indicated when the frequency of breakdown to a manifest exotropia is significant. Even if the girl had been seen and diagnosed with it when she was three, she may not have needed surgery at that point in time. Does that make the GP not liable?

Assuming that a body of responsible and reputable medical professionals agree that surgery might not have been an option for a three-year-old girl, the GP may not be liable for negligence even if he failed to exclude (or mention his inability to exclude) the latent exophoria. Also note the latest English case of *Chester v Afshar* (see Appendix 3).

Failure to Inform a Patient of Ocular Side Effects of Steroids – Medical Negligence in Informed Consent

A young patient with eczema has been seeing his regular general practitioner (GP) who has been treating his condition with topical steroids for many years. The patient experiences deteriorating vision and goes to see an ophthalmologist who diagnoses him with having steroid induced cataract and glaucoma.

(a) Is the GP liable? If he had told his patient about the possible ocular side effects of steroids but did not refer him to an ophthalmologist, is he still liable?

(b) The GP did not tell his patient about the specific ocular side effects of steroids but did refer him to an ophthalmologist many years ago (before the patient had any vision symptoms). The patient missed the appointment. The GP did not follow up with the patient on this matter, and assumed that he had seen an ophthalmologist and would be under his care. Is the GP still liable?

Answers

(a) Is the GP liable? If he had told his patient about the possible ocular side effects of steroids but did not refer him to an ophthalmologist, is he still liable?

The GP must obtain proper consent from his patient by informing him of the side effects of topical steroids. It is the medical duty of care of a doctor to advise his patient about the risks and side effects of medications. Under the *Bolam* test, if it is the accepted current practice to inform a patient of steroid induced cataract and glaucoma, which the above GP had failed to do, then he could be liable for negligence. Whether the GP is liable for failing to refer the patient to an ophthalmologist will depend on whether it is the accepted current practice to refer a patient at that point of time. The *Bolam* test applies.

(b) The GP did not tell his patient about the specific ocular side effects of steroids but did refer him to an ophthalmologist many years ago (before the patient had any vision symptoms). The patient missed the appointment. The GP did not follow up with the patient on this matter, and assumed that he had seen an ophthalmologist and would be under his care. Is the GP still liable?

If the GP can show that the patient's failure to keep the appointment with the ophthalmologist broke the link between his substandard advice and the patient's final condition, the GP can escape liability. In other words, the GP can argue that even if he has failed to counsel the patient adequately, any responsible and competent ophthalmologist will have done so. This would have happened if the patient had kept the appointment. By missing the appointment, the patient himself missed the opportunity to obtain proper advice, breaking the link between the GP's substandard advice and the final outcome.

Take-home Message

It is important to warn patients of side-effects of treatment given.

Case Scenario 35

Patient with a History of Epilepsy — Should the Doctor Report?

A doctor attends to a patient with a history of epilepsy who has been involved in a traffic accident; the patient is a driver.

Should the doctor report this to the Land Transport Authority?

Answers

Should the doctor report this to the Land Transport Authority?

Every doctor has a duty of confidentiality to his patients. These duties of confidentiality are found in the codes of ethics and the law.

> *The Hippocratic Oath*
> … Whatever, in connection with my professional service, or not in connection with it, I see or hear, in the life of men, which ought not to be spoken of abroad, I will not divulge, as reckoning that all such should be kept secret.

> In the case of *Hunter v Mann*:
> … The doctor is under a duty not to disclose (voluntarily) without the consent of his patient information which he, the doctor, has obtained in his professional capacity, save in very exceptional circumstances.

Medical ethics justifies the respect for the autonomy of the individual and the patient's privacy rights. There is a clear public interest to maintain medical confidence. The confidentiality of a patient's relationship with his doctor is fundamental to ethical medical practice. The ethical duty to maintain medical confidentiality allows patients to discuss their health with their doctors freely, safe in the knowledge that there is patient confidentiality. Any doctor found breaching this patient confidentiality may be subject to disciplinary action by the medical profession. The patient is protected from harm that may result from an unauthorized disclosure of information.

Under the common law, a doctor's duty of care to his patient includes a duty not to give a third party a certificate as to his patient's condition. Hence, a patient can sue for medical negligence if he has been harmed physically by the improper disclosure of medical information as seen in *Furniss v Fitchett* (1958).

However, a patient's medical information may be disclosed under certain circumstances. To depart from the general rule of patient confidentiality, consideration will be given to the reasonable professional conduct that is appropriate in the circumstances of a particular case.

The exceptions to the duty of confidentiality are made when

- a patient consents to the disclosure
- it is in compliance with statutory notification under the Infectious Diseases Act

- it is in compliance with a court order
- it is in communication with other doctors on treatment
- disclosure is in the public interest

In this case, if the doctor is of the opinion that the patient's condition may endanger his own life as well as that of other road users, then the doctor may disclose it to the Land Transport Authority because it is in the public interest to disclose such information under the limits or exceptions of confidentiality.

Appendix 1

The *Bolam* Case

Bolam v Friern Hospital Management Committee (1957) **1 WLR 582**

The plaintiff patient was suffering from mental illness and had to undergo electroconvulsive therapy (ECT). He had not given informed consent. During the ECT, he was not given any relaxant drugs and was also largely unrestrained. The patient sustained dislocation of both hip joints and fractures of the pelvis.

The court held that the doctors did not breach their duty when deciding against restraining the patient. McHair J said:

> Where you get a situation which involves the use of some special skill or competence, then the test as to whether there has been negligence or not is not the test of the man on the top of a Clapham omnibus, because he has not got this special skill. The test is the standard of the ordinary skilled man exercising and professing to have that special skill. A man need not possess the highest expert skill: it is well-established law that it is sufficient if he exercises the ordinary skill of an ordinary competent man exercising that particular art.

The *Bolam* Test

The *Bolam* case considered that the standard of care was that of professional colleagues, which must accord with a "responsible body of medical opinion". The doctor is not measured by the standard of the reasonable man in the street but by the standard of the reasonable doctor. In deciding whether a doctor is negligent, the court will rely on the expert professional opinion. Under the *Bolam* test, a doctor is not negligent if he has conformed with responsible professional practices.

Appendix 2

The *Bolitho* Case

Bolitho v Hackney Health Authority (1997) 4 All 771

P, a two-year-old boy, who had a history of hospital treatment for croup, was readmitted to hospital under the care of two doctors, Dr H and Dr R. The following day, P suffered two short episodes at 12.30 p.m. and 2 p.m. during which he turned white and had difficulty breathing. Dr H was called in the first instance; in the second instance, she delegated to Dr R to attend to P. However, neither doctor attended to P, who at both times appeared to return quickly to a stable condition.

At around 2.30 p.m., P suffered total respiratory failure and a cardiac arrest resulting in severe brain damage. P died later. P's mother as the administratrix of P's estate sued for medical negligence. The defendant health authority accepted that Dr H had breached her duty of care to P, but alleged that the cardiac arrest could not have been avoided even if Dr H had attended to P earlier than 2.30 p.m.

It was known that intubation to provide an airway would have ensured that respiratory failure did not lead to a cardiac arrest and that such intubation should have been carried out after the first episode.

P's lawyer had expert evidence that a reasonably competent doctor would have intubated the patient in such circumstances. The defendant doctor had her own expert witness (Dr D) to say that non-intubation was a clinically justifiable response.

The High Court judge found that the views of the two experts, though diametrically opposed, represented a responsible body of professional opinion espoused by distinguished and truth experts.

The court held that Dr H, if she had attended to P and not intubated him, would have met the standard of a proper level of skill and competence according to Dr D's views, and that it had not been proven that the defendants' admitted breach of duty **caused the injury** to P. The Court of Appeal dismissed an appeal by P's mother, who later appealed to the House of Lords.

The House of Lords held that a doctor could be liable for negligence in respect to diagnosis and treatment despite a body of professional opinion sanctioning his conduct, where it had not been shown to the judge's satisfaction that the body of opinion relied on was **reasonable** or **responsible**.

In most cases, the fact that distinguished experts in the field were of a particular opinion showed the reasonableness of that opinion. However, in a rare case, if it could be demonstrated that the professional opinion was not capable of withstanding logical analysis, the judge could hold that the body of opinion was not reasonable or responsible. As the House of Lords accepted Dr D's views as reasonable, the appeal was thus dismissed.

The *Bolitho* Test

The body of opinion relied upon must have a **basis in logic**, and the judge must be satisfied that the experts have directed their minds to the question of **comparative risks and benefits**, and have reached a defensible conclusion on the matter.

Under the *Bolam* test, a doctor is not negligent if what he has done is accepted by a responsible body of medical opinion. But the court must be satisfied that the **body of opinion rests on a logical basis**.

Appendix 3

The *Chester v Afshar* Case

Chester v Afshar (2005) Lloyds L.R. 109

The recent English case of *Chester v Afshar* alters the law on informed consent. The defendant neurosurgeon had performed surgery on the patient plaintiff who was suffering from low back pain. Her consultant rheumatologist had given her epidural and sclerosant injections. An MRI scan showed disc protusions. She was referred to a neurosurgeon for elective lumbar surgical procedure. Prior to the surgery, the defendant neurosurgeon had negligently failed to warn the patient plaintiff of the small 1–2% risks of *cauda equine* syndrome (CES). The patient had a discectomy to treat her low back pain. The surgeon performed the procedure competently without negligence. Unfortunately, the patient suffered *cauda equine* damage as an unavoidable complication of this surgery, and subsequent disability. She sued the surgeon claiming that he failed to warn her about this particular risk.

As the surgeon lacked documentary evidence that he had warned the patient of CES risk, the court accepted the patient's allegation, and liability for failure to warn was established. Under traditional causation principles, the next step was to convince the court that the patient would not have undergone the procedure had she been aware of the risk (i.e. causation). The patient, however, took a different approach in this case. She agreed that she might still have had the surgery after being warned about the risk, but added that she would have taken time to think about it and schedule the surgery for another day, possibly by a different surgeon.

Thus, had an appropriate warning of the risk of *cauda equine* damage been given by the surgeon, the patient would not then have agreed to surgery on that day, but would have taken further opinion as to whether surgery was necessary.

Lord Hoffman said that it "was about as logical as saying that if one had been told, on entering a casino, that the odds on No. 7 coming up at roulette were only 1 in 37, one would have gone away and come back next week or gone to a different casino".

By a majority, the judges found that the patient had established a causal link between the breach (i.e. failure to warn of CES risk) and the injury (i.e. nerve damage) the patient had sustained, and held that the surgeon was liable for damages. But for the surgeon's negligent failure to warn the patient of the small risk of serious injury, the actual injury would not have occurred when it did and the chance of it occurring on a subsequent occasion was very small. The patient's injury was the product of the very risk that the patient should have been warned about when she gave her consent. As a result of the surgeon's failure to warn the patient, the patient could not be said to have given informed consent to the surgery in the full legal sense.

The court took the view that the negligence to inform of risk that led to injury was satisfied on policy grounds, the policy being that the patient's autonomy and dignity should be respected by allowing her to make an informed decision.

The patient's right of autonomy and dignity could and should be vindicated by a narrow and modest departure from traditional causation principles. Thus, legally, the patient's injury was considered to have been caused by the breach of the surgeon's duty of medical care that prevented the patient from giving a proper informed consent.

The implication of the new ruling of the *Chester* case now makes it more important than ever to take extreme care in ensuring that patients, including human subjects in clinical trials, are fully informed, that they understand the information given to them, and that they are given sufficient time to digest the information. Careful and comprehensible warnings about all significant possible adverse outcomes must be given.

Appendix 4

The Road Traffic Act

PART IV
GENERAL PROVISIONS RELATING TO ROAD TRAFFIC

Division 1 – Provisions as to driving and offences in connection therewith

Restriction on driving by young persons

62.   (1) A person below the age of 18 years shall not drive a motor vehicle on a road.
[1/99]

(2) A person who has attained the age of 18 years but who is below the age of 21 years shall not drive a heavy locomotive, light locomotive, motor tractor or heavy motor car on a road.
[11/96]

(3) The burden of establishing his age shall rest on the applicant for a driving licence.

(4) A person who drives or causes or permits any person to drive a motor vehicle in contravention of this section shall be guilty of an offence.

(5) A person prohibited by this section by reason of his age from driving a motor vehicle or a motor vehicle of any class shall, for the purposes of Part II, be deemed to be disqualified under the provisions of that Part from holding or obtaining any licence other than a licence to drive such motor vehicles, if any, as he is not by this section forbidden to drive.

Restriction on driving certain categories of heavy motor vehicles

62A. A person who has attained the age of 70 years shall not drive a vehicle belonging to the following categories or classes of motor vehicles:

(a) heavy locomotives;
(b) light locomotives;
(c) motor tractors; and
(d) heavy motor cars.
[7/90; 21/2002]

Rate of speed

63. (1) Except as otherwise provided by this Act, it shall not be lawful for any person to drive a motor vehicle of any class or description on a road at a speed greater than any speed which may be prescribed as the maximum speed in relation to a vehicle of that class or description.

(2) The Minister may, by notification in the Gazette, prohibit the driving of motor vehicles generally or of particular classes of motor vehicles above a specified speed over any specified road or part of a specified road either generally or for a specified time or times.

(3) So long as any prohibition made under subsection (2) remains in force, the Minister may cause or permit to be placed or erected and maintained traffic signs which shall state the substance of the notification in the Gazette containing the prohibition and which shall be placed in such positions as shall give adequate notice thereof to drivers of motor vehicles.

(4) A person who drives a motor vehicle on a road at a speed exceeding any speed limit imposed by or in exercise of powers conferred by this Act shall be guilty of an offence.

Reckless or dangerous driving

64. (1) If any person drives a motor vehicle on a road recklessly, or at a speed or in a manner which is dangerous to the public, having regard to all the circumstances of the case, including the nature, condition and use of the road, and the amount of traffic which is actually at the time, or which might reasonably be expected to be, on the road, he shall be guilty of an offence and shall be liable on conviction to a fine not exceeding $3,000 or to imprisonment for a term not exceeding 12 months or to both and, in the case of a second or subsequent conviction, to a fine not exceeding $5,000 or to imprisonment for a term not exceeding 2 years or to both.
[11/96]

(2) On a second or subsequent conviction under this section, the convicting court shall exercise the power conferred by section 42 of ordering that the offender shall be disqualified from holding or obtaining a driving licence unless the court, having regard to the lapse of time since the date of the previous or last previous conviction or for any other special reason, thinks fit to order otherwise.

(3) Subsection (2) shall not be construed as affecting the right of the court to exercise the power under section 42 on a first conviction.
S 304/2005, wef 17/05/2005

(4) Where a person is convicted of abetting the commission of an offence under this section and it is proved that he was present in the motor vehicle at the time of the commission of the offence, the offence of which he is convicted shall, for the purpose of the provisions of Part II relating to disqualification from holding or obtaining driving licences, be deemed to be an offence in connection with the driving of a motor vehicle.

(5) Any police officer may arrest without warrant any person committing an offence under this section.
[1/99]

Driving without due care or reasonable consideration

65. If any person drives a motor vehicle on a road –

(a) without due care and attention; or

(b) without reasonable consideration for other persons using the road,

he shall be guilty of an offence and shall be liable on conviction to a fine not exceeding $1,000 or to imprisonment for a term not exceeding 6 months or to both and, in the case of a second or subsequent conviction, to a fine not exceeding $2,000 or to imprisonment for a term not exceeding 12 months or to both.
[11/96]

Collision of heavy motor vehicles and public service vehicles with buildings or structures

65A. (1) Any person who, when driving or attempting to drive –

(a) a heavy motor vehicle as defined in section 79 (6); or

(b) any public service vehicle which is classified as a type of bus under the Second Schedule,

causes the heavy motor vehicle or public service vehicle to collide with any building or structure shall be guilty of an offence and shall be liable on conviction to a fine not exceeding $5,000 or to imprisonment for a term not exceeding 2 years or to both and, in the case of a second or subsequent conviction, to a fine not exceeding $10,000 or to imprisonment for a term not exceeding 5 years or to both.
[11/96; 28/2001]

(1A) The Minister may, by notification in the Gazette, prescribe particulars of any structure including its location and maximum headroom measurement.
[Act 4/2006, wef 27/02/2006]

(2) In this section, "structure" includes any bus shelter, gantry post, overhead bridge and pillar.
[11/96]

Use of mobile telephone while driving

65B. (1) Any person who, being the driver of a motor vehicle on a road or in a public place, uses a mobile telephone while the motor vehicle is in motion shall be guilty of an offence and shall be liable on conviction to a fine not exceeding $1,000 or to imprisonment for a term not exceeding 6 months or to both, and, in the case of a second or subsequent conviction, to a fine not exceeding $2,000 or to imprisonment for a term not exceeding 12 months or to both.
[1/99]

(2) In this section –

"mobile telephone" includes any hand held equipment which is designed or capable of being used for telecommunication;

"use", in relation to a mobile telephone, means to hold it in one hand while using it to communicate with any person.

[1/99]

Causing death by reckless or dangerous driving

66. (1) Any person who causes the death of another person by the driving of a motor vehicle on a road recklessly, or at a speed or in a manner which is dangerous to the public, having regard to all the circumstances of the case, including the nature, condition and use of the road, and the amount of traffic which is actually at the time, or which might reasonably be expected to be, on the road, shall be guilty of an offence and shall be liable on conviction to imprisonment for a term not exceeding 5 years.

(2) Section 280 of the Criminal Procedure Code (Cap. 68) shall apply to any offence under this section as it applies to the offence of causing death by a rash or negligent act.

(3) If upon the trial of a person for an offence under this section the court is not satisfied that his driving was the cause of the death, but is satisfied that he is guilty of driving as specified in subsection (1), it shall be lawful for the court to convict him of an offence under section 64, whether or not the requirements of section 82 have been satisfied as respects that offence.

Driving while under influence of drink or drugs

67. (1) Any person who, when driving or attempting to drive a motor vehicle on a road or other public place –

(a) is unfit to drive in that he is under the influence of drink or of a drug or an intoxicating substance to such an extent as to be incapable of having proper control of such vehicle; or

(b) has so much alcohol in his body that the proportion of it in his breath or blood exceeds the prescribed limit,

shall be guilty of an offence and shall be liable on conviction to a fine of not less than $1,000 and not more than $5,000 or to imprisonment for a term not exceeding 6 months and, in the case of a second or subsequent conviction, to a fine of not less than $3,000 and not more than $10,000 and to imprisonment for a term not exceeding 12 months.

[11/96]

(2) A person convicted of an offence under this section shall, unless the court for special reasons thinks fit to order otherwise and without prejudice to the power of the court to order a longer period of disqualification, be disqualified from holding or obtaining a driving licence for a period of not less than 12 months from the date of his conviction or, where he is sentenced to imprisonment, from the date of his release from prison.

[7/90]

(3) Any police officer may arrest without warrant any person committing an offence under this section.
[7/90]

Enhanced penalties for offenders with previous convictions under certain sections

67A. (1) Where a person having been convicted on at least 2 previous occasions of any one or more of the offences under sections 43 (4), 47 (5), 47C (7), 63 (4), 64 (1), 66 (1), 67 (1) and 70 (4) is again convicted of an offence under sections 43 (4), 47 (5), 47C (7), 63 (4), 64 (1), 66 (1), 67 (1) or 70 (4), the court shall have the power to impose a punishment in excess of that prescribed for such conviction as follows:

(a) where the court is satisfied, by reason of his previous convictions or his antecedents, that it is expedient for the protection of the public or with the view to the prevention of further commission of any such offence that a punishment in excess of that prescribed for such a conviction should be awarded, then the court may punish such offender with punishment not exceeding 3 times the amount of punishment to which he would otherwise have been liable for such a conviction except that where imprisonment is imposed it shall not exceed 10 years; and

(b) notwithstanding section 11 of the Criminal Procedure Code (Cap. 68), if –

(i) such offender, while committing the offence under sections 43 (4), 47 (5), 47C (7), 63 (4), 64 (1), 66 (1) or 67 (1) causes any serious injury or death to another person; or

(ii) in the case of an offender under section 70 (4), such offender had, in driving or attempting to drive a motor vehicle at the time of any accident leading to his arrest under section 69 (5), caused any serious injury or death to another person, the court may also punish him, subject to section 231 of the Criminal Procedure Code, with caning with not more than 6 strokes.
[11/96; 1/99]

(2) This section shall not apply to a person who has been convicted of an offence under section 63 (4) unless the court is satisfied that in committing such offence and the offence in respect of which he had been previously convicted, he had driven a motor vehicle on a road at a speed which exceeded by 40 kilometres per hour the speed limit imposed by or in exercise of powers conferred by this Act.
[11/96]

(3) In subsection (1), "serious injury" has the same meaning as in section 47D.

(4) Notwithstanding any provision to the contrary in the Criminal Procedure Code, a District Court or Magistrate's Court may award the full punishment prescribed by this section.

Being in charge of motor vehicle when under influence of drink or drugs

68. (1) Any person who when in charge of a motor vehicle which is on a road or other public place but not driving the vehicle –

(a) is unfit to drive in that he is under the influence of drink or of a drug or an intoxicating substance to such an extent as to be incapable of having proper control of a vehicle; or

(b) has so much alcohol in his body that the proportion of it in his breath or blood exceeds the prescribed limit,

shall be guilty of an offence and shall be liable on conviction to a fine of not less than $500 and not more than $2,000 or to imprisonment for a term not exceeding 3 months and, in the case of a second or subsequent conviction, to a fine of not less than $1,000 and not more than $5,000 and to imprisonment for a term not exceeding 6 months.
[11/96]

(2) For the purpose of subsection (1), a person shall be deemed not to have been in charge of a motor vehicle if he proves –

(a) that at the material time the circumstances were such that there was no likelihood of his driving the vehicle so long as he remained so unfit to drive or so long as the proportion of alcohol in his breath or blood remained in excess of the prescribed limit; and
(b) that between his becoming so unfit to drive and the material time, or between the time when the proportion of alcohol in his breath or blood first exceeded the prescribed limit and the material time, he had not driven the vehicle on a road or other public place.
[11/96]

(3) On a second or subsequent conviction for an offence under this section, the offender shall, unless the court for special reasons thinks fit to order otherwise and without prejudice to the power of the court to order a longer period of disqualification, be disqualified from holding or obtaining a driving licence for a period of 12 months from the date of his release from prison.
[7/90]

(4) Where a person convicted of an offence under this section has been previously convicted of an offence under section 67, he shall be treated for the purpose of this section as having been previously convicted under this section.
[7/90]

(5) Any police officer may arrest without warrant any person committing an offence under this section.
[7/90]

Breath tests

69.   (1) Where a police officer has reasonable cause to suspect that –

(a) a person driving or attempting to drive or in charge of a motor vehicle on a road or other public place has alcohol in his body or has committed a traffic offence whilst the vehicle was in motion;
(b) a person has been driving or attempting to drive or been in charge of a motor vehicle on a road or other public place with alcohol in his body and that he still has alcohol in his body;

(c) a person has been driving or attempting to drive or been in charge of a motor vehicle on a road or other public place and has committed a traffic offence whilst the vehicle was in motion; or

(d) a person has been driving or attempting to drive or been in charge of a motor vehicle on a road or other public place when an accident occurred –

(i) between that motor vehicle and one or more other motor vehicles; or
(ii) causing any injury or death to another person,

the police officer may, subject to section 71, require that person to provide a specimen of his breath for a breath test.
[11/96]

(2) A person may be required under subsection (1) to provide a specimen of his breath either at or near the place where the requirement is made or, if the requirement is made under subsection (1) (d) and the police officer making the requirement thinks fit, at a police station specified by the police officer.
[11/96]

(3) A breath test required under subsection (1) shall be conducted by a police officer.
[11/96]

(4) A person who fails, without reasonable excuse, to provide a specimen of his breath when required to do so in pursuance of this section shall be guilty of an offence and shall be liable on conviction to a fine of not less than $1,000 and not more than $5,000 or to imprisonment for a term not exceeding 6 months and, in the case of a second or subsequent conviction, to a fine of not less than $3,000 and not more than $10,000 and to imprisonment for a term not exceeding 12 months.
[11/96]

(5) A police officer may arrest a person without warrant if –

(a) as a result of a breath test he has reasonable cause to suspect that the proportion of alcohol in that person's breath or blood exceeds the prescribed limit;
(b) that person has failed to provide a specimen of his breath for a breath test when required to do so in pursuance of this section and the police officer has reasonable cause to suspect that he has alcohol in his body; or
(c) he has reasonable cause to suspect that that person is under the influence of a drug or an intoxicating substance.

(6) A person shall not be arrested by virtue of subsection (5) when he is at a hospital as a patient.
[11/96]

Provision of specimen for analysis

70. (1) In the course of an investigation whether a person arrested under section 69 (5) has committed an offence under section 67 or 68, a police officer may, subject to the provisions of this section and section 71, require him –

(a) to provide a specimen of his breath for analysis by means of a prescribed breath alcohol analyser; or

(b) to provide at a hospital a specimen of his blood for a laboratory test,

notwithstanding that he has been required to provide a specimen of his breath for a breath test under section 69 (1).
[11/96]

(2) A breath test under this section shall be conducted by a police officer and shall only be conducted at a police station.
[11/96]

(3) A requirement under this section to provide a specimen of blood –

(a) shall not be made unless –

(i) the police officer making the requirement has reasonable cause to believe that for medical reasons a specimen of breath cannot be provided or should not be required;

(ii) at the time the requirement is made, the prescribed breath alcohol analyser is not available at the police station or it is for any other reason not practicable to use the breath alcohol analyser; or

(iii) the police officer making the requirement has reasonable cause to suspect that the person required to provide the specimen is under the influence of a drug or an intoxicating substance; and

(b) may be made notwithstanding that the person required to provide the specimen has already provided or been required to provide a specimen of his breath.
[11/96]

(4) A person who fails, without reasonable excuse, to provide a specimen when required to do so in pursuance of this section shall be guilty of an offence and if it is shown that at the time of any accident referred to in section 69 (1) (d) or of his arrest under section 69 (5) –

(a) he was driving or attempting to drive a motor vehicle on a road or any other public place, he shall be liable on conviction to be punished as if the offence charged were an offence under section 67; or

(b) he was in charge of a motor vehicle on a road or any other public place, he shall be liable on conviction to be punished as if the offence charged were an offence under section 68.
[11/96]

(5) A police officer shall, on requiring any person under this section to provide a specimen for a laboratory test, warn him that failure to provide a specimen of blood may make him liable to imprisonment, a fine and disqualification, and, if the police officer fails to do so, the court before which that person is charged with an offence under subsection (4) may dismiss the charge.
[11/96]

Protection of hospital patients

71.   (1) A person who is at a hospital as a patient shall not be required to provide a specimen for a breath test or to provide a specimen for a laboratory test unless the medical practitioner in immediate charge of his case authorises it and the specimen is to be provided at the hospital.
[11/96]

(2) The medical practitioner referred to in subsection (1) shall not authorise a specimen to be taken where it would be prejudicial to the proper care and treatment of the patient.
[11/96]

Evidence in proceedings for offences under sections 67 and 68

71A. (1) In proceedings for an offence under section 67 or 68, evidence of the proportion of alcohol or of any drug or intoxicating substance in a specimen of breath or blood (as the case may be) provided by the accused shall be taken into account and, subject to subsection (2), it shall be assumed that the proportion of alcohol in the accused's breath or blood at the time of the alleged offence was not less than in the specimen.
[11/96]

(2) Where the proceedings are for an offence under section 67 (1) (a) or 68 (1) (a) and it is alleged that, at the time of the offence, the accused was unfit to drive in that he was under the influence of drink, or for an offence under section 67 (1) (b) or 68 (1) (b), the assumption referred to in subsection (1) shall not be made if the accused proves –

(a) that he consumed alcohol after he had ceased to drive, attempt to drive or be in charge of a motor vehicle on a road or any other public place and before he provided the specimen; and
(b) that had he not done so the proportion of alcohol in his breath or blood –

(i) would not have been such as to make him unfit to drive a motor vehicle in the case of proceedings for an offence under section 67 (1) (a) or 68 (1) (a); or
(ii) would not have exceeded the prescribed limit in the case of proceedings for an offence under section 67 (1) (b) or 68 (1) (b).
[11/96]

(3) Subject to subsection (5) –

(a) evidence of the proportion of alcohol in a specimen of breath may be given by the production of a document or documents purporting to be either a statement automatically produced by a prescribed breath alcohol analyser and a certificate signed by a police officer (which may but need not be contained in the same document as the statement) to the effect that the statement relates to a specimen provided by the accused at the date and time shown in the statement; and

(b) evidence of the proportion of alcohol or of any drug or intoxicating substance in a specimen of blood may be given by the production of a document purporting to be a certificate signed by an authorised analyst as to the proportion of alcohol, drug or intoxicating substance found in a specimen of blood identified in the certificate.
[11/96]

(4) A specimen of blood shall be disregarded unless it was taken from the accused with his consent by a medical practitioner; but evidence that a specimen of blood was so taken may be given by the production of a document purporting to certify that fact and to be signed by a medical practitioner.
[11/96]

(5) A document purporting to be such a statement or such a certificate, or both, as is mentioned in subsection (3) is admissible in evidence on behalf of the prosecution in pursuance of this section only if a copy of it has been handed to the accused when the document was produced or has been served on him not later than 7 days before the hearing, and any other document is so admissible only if a copy of it has been served on the accused not later than 7 days before the hearing.
[11/96]

(6) A document purporting to be a certificate (or so much of a document as purports to be a certificate) is not so admissible if the accused, not later than 3 days before the hearing or within such further time as the court may in special circumstances allow, has served notice on the prosecution requiring the attendance at the hearing of the person by whom the document purports to be signed.
[11/96]

(7) A copy of a certificate required by this section to be served on the accused or a notice required by this section to be served on the prosecution may be served personally or sent by registered post.
[11/96]

Deputy Commissioner of Police may require medical practitioner to send blood specimen for laboratory test

71B. (1) Notwithstanding anything in section 69 or 71A, where a person –

(a) was the driver of or attempted to drive or was in charge of a motor vehicle on a road or other public place when an accident occurred –

(i) between that motor vehicle and one or more other motor vehicles; or
(ii) causing any injury or death to another person; and

(b) as a result of any injury sustained by him in the accident or any other cause is unable to provide a specimen of his breath under section 69 or to give his consent to a specimen of blood being taken from him for analysis,

any medical practitioner treating such person for his injury shall, if so directed by the Deputy Commissioner of Police, cause any specimen of blood taken by the medical practitioner from such person in connection with his treatment to be sent for a laboratory test to determine the proportion of alcohol or of any drug or intoxicating substance in the specimen.
[11/96]

(2) In proceedings for an offence under section 67 or 68, evidence of the proportion of alcohol or of any drug or intoxicating substance in a specimen of blood analysed in pursuance of this section shall be taken into account.
[11/96]

(3) Evidence of the proportion of alcohol or of any drug or intoxicating substance in a specimen of blood analysed under this section may, subject to subsection (4), be given by the production of a document purporting to be a certificate signed by an authorised analyst as to the proportion of alcohol, drug or intoxicating substance found in the specimen of blood identified in the certificate.
[11/96]

(4) The provisions of section 71A (5), (6) and (7) shall apply, with the necessary modifications, to a certificate referred to in subsection (3) as they apply to a document or certificate referred to in section 71A (3).
[11/96]

Interpretation of sections 67 to 71B
72.   (1) In sections 67 to 71B –

"authorised analyst" means any medical practitioner, scientific officer or chemist who is employed in a hospital or laboratory to carry out analyses of blood;
"breath test" means a test for the purpose of obtaining, by means of a breath alcohol analyser or any other device prescribed by the Minister, an indication whether the proportion of alcohol in a person's breath or blood is likely to exceed the prescribed limit;
"fail" includes refuse;
"intoxicating substance" has the same meaning as in the Intoxicating Substances Act (Cap. 146A);
"police station" includes any place or conveyance authorised or appointed by the Deputy Commissioner of Police to be used as a police station;
"prescribed limit" means –

(a) 35 microgrammes of alcohol in 100 millilitres of breath; or
(b) 80 milligrammes of alcohol in 100 millilitres of blood.
[11/96; 1/99]

(2) A person does not provide a specimen of breath for a breath test or for analysis unless the specimen is sufficient to enable the test or the analysis to be carried out and is provided in such a way as to enable the objective of the test or analysis to be satisfactorily achieved.
[11/96]

(3) Subject to section 71B, a person provides a specimen of blood if and only if he consents to its being taken by a medical practitioner and it is so taken.
[11/96]

Appendix 5

The Declaration of Helsinki

WORLD MEDICAL ASSOCIATION DECLARATION OF HELSINKI
Ethical Principles for Medical Research Involving Human Subjects
Adopted by the 18th WMA General Assembly, Helsinki, Finland, June 1964, and amended by the
29th WMA General Assembly, Tokyo, Japan, October 1975
35th WMA General Assembly, Venice, Italy, October 1983
41st WMA General Assembly, Hong Kong, September 1989
48th WMA General Assembly, Somerset West, Republic of South Africa, October 1996
and the 52nd WMA General Assembly, Edinburgh, Scotland, October 2000
Note of Clarification on Paragraph 29 added by the WMA General Assembly, Washington 2002
Note of Clarification on Paragraph 30 added by the WMA General Assembly, Tokyo 2004

A. INTRODUCTION

1.   The World Medical Association has developed the Declaration of Helsinki as a statement of
     ethical principles to provide guidance to physicians and other participants in medical research
     involving human subjects. Medical research involving human subjects includes research on
     identifiable human material or identifiable data.

2.   It is the duty of the physician to promote and safeguard the health of the people. The
     physician's knowledge and conscience are dedicated to the fulfillment of this duty.

3.   The Declaration of Geneva of the World Medical Association binds the physician with the
     words, "The health of my patient will be my first consideration," and the International Code
     of Medical Ethics declares that, "A physician shall act only in the patient's interest when
     providing medical care which might have the effect of weakening the physical and mental
     condition of the patient."

---

4. Medical progress is based on research which ultimately must rest in part on experimentation involving human subjects.

5. In medical research on human subjects, considerations related to the well-being of the human subject should take precedence over the interests of science and society.

6. The primary purpose of medical research involving human subjects is to improve prophylactic, diagnostic and therapeutic procedures and the understanding of the aetiology and pathogenesis of disease. Even the best proven prophylactic, diagnostic, and therapeutic methods must continuously be challenged through research for their effectiveness, efficiency, accessibility and quality.

7. In current medical practice and in medical research, most prophylactic, diagnostic and therapeutic procedures involve risks and burdens.

8. Medical research is subject to ethical standards that promote respect for all human beings and protect their health and rights. Some research populations are vulnerable and need special protection. The particular needs of the economically and medically disadvantaged must be recognized. Special attention is also required for those who cannot give or refuse consent for themselves, for those who may be subject to giving consent under duress, for those who will not benefit personally from the research and for those for whom the research is combined with care.

9. Research Investigators should be aware of the ethical, legal and regulatory requirements for research on human subjects in their own countries as well as applicable international requirements. No national ethical, legal or regulatory requirement should be allowed to reduce or eliminate any of the protections for human subjects set forth in this Declaration.

B. BASIC PRINCIPLES FOR ALL MEDICAL RESEARCH

10. It is the duty of the physician in medical research to protect the life, health, privacy, and dignity of the human subject.

11. Medical research involving human subjects must conform to generally accepted scientific principles, be based on a thorough knowledge of the scientific literature, other relevant sources of information, and on adequate laboratory and, where appropriate, animal experimentation.

12. Appropriate caution must be exercised in the conduct of research which may affect the environment, and the welfare of animals used for research must be respected.

13. The design and performance of each experimental procedure involving human subjects should be clearly formulated in an experimental protocol. This protocol should be submitted for consideration, comment, guidance, and where appropriate, approval to a specially appointed ethical review committee, which must be independent of the investigator, the sponsor or any other kind of undue influence. This independent committee should be in conformity with the laws and regulations of the country in which the research experiment is performed. The

committee has the right to monitor ongoing trials. The researcher has the obligation to provide monitoring information to the committee, especially any serious adverse events. The researcher should also submit to the committee, for review, information regarding funding, sponsors, institutional affiliations, other potential conflicts of interest and incentives for subjects.

14.   The research protocol should always contain a statement of the ethical considerations involved and should indicate that there is compliance with the principles enunciated in this Declaration.

15.   Medical research involving human subjects should be conducted only by scientifically qualified persons and under the supervision of a clinically competent medical person. The responsibility for the human subject must always rest with a medically qualified person and never rest on the subject of the research, even though the subject has given consent.

16.   Every medical research project involving human subjects should be preceded by careful assessment of predictable risks and burdens in comparison with foreseeable benefits to the subject or to others. This does not preclude the participation of healthy volunteers in medical research. The design of all studies should be publicly available.

17.   Physicians should abstain from engaging in research projects involving human subjects unless they are confident that the risks involved have been adequately assessed and can be satisfactorily managed. Physicians should cease any investigation if the risks are found to outweigh the potential benefits or if there is conclusive proof of positive and beneficial results.

18.   Medical research involving human subjects should only be conducted if the importance of the objective outweighs the inherent risks and burdens to the subject. This is especially important when the human subjects are healthy volunteers.

19.   Medical research is only justified if there is a reasonable likelihood that the populations in which the research is carried out stand to benefit from the results of the research.

20.   The subjects must be volunteers and informed participants in the research project.

21.   The right of research subjects to safeguard their integrity must always be respected. Every precaution should be taken to respect the privacy of the subject, the confidentiality of the patient's information and to minimize the impact of the study on the subject's physical and mental integrity and on the personality of the subject.

22.   In any research on human beings, each potential subject must be adequately informed of the aims, methods, sources of funding, any possible conflicts of interest, institutional affiliations of the researcher, the anticipated benefits and potential risks of the study and the discomfort it may entail. The subject should be informed of the right to abstain from participation in the study or to withdraw consent to participate at any time without reprisal. After ensuring that the subject has understood the information, the physician should then obtain the subject's freely-given informed consent, preferably in writing. If the consent cannot be obtained in writing, the non-written consent must be formally documented and witnessed.

23. When obtaining informed consent for the research project the physician should be particularly cautious if the subject is in a dependent relationship with the physician or may consent under duress. In that case the informed consent should be obtained by a well-informed physician who is not engaged in the investigation and who is completely independent of this relationship.

24. For a research subject who is legally incompetent, physically or mentally incapable of giving consent or is a legally incompetent minor, the investigator must obtain informed consent from the legally authorized representative in accordance with applicable law. These groups should not be included in research unless the research is necessary to promote the health of the population represented and this research cannot instead be performed on legally competent persons.

25. When a subject deemed legally incompetent, such as a minor child, is able to give assent to decisions about participation in research, the investigator must obtain that assent in addition to the consent of the legally authorized representative.

26. Research on individuals from whom it is not possible to obtain consent, including proxy or advance consent, should be done only if the physical/mental condition that prevents obtaining informed consent is a necessary characteristic of the research population. The specific reasons for involving research subjects with a condition that renders them unable to give informed consent should be stated in the experimental protocol for consideration and approval of the review committee. The protocol should state that consent to remain in the research should be obtained as soon as possible from the individual or a legally authorized surrogate.

27. Both authors and publishers have ethical obligations. In publication of the results of research, the investigators are obliged to preserve the accuracy of the results. Negative as well as positive results should be published or otherwise publicly available. Sources of funding, institutional affiliations and any possible conflicts of interest should be declared in the publication. Reports of experimentation not in accordance with the principles laid down in this Declaration should not be accepted for publication.

C. ADDITIONAL PRINCIPLES FOR MEDICAL RESEARCH COMBINED WITH MEDICAL CARE

28. The physician may combine medical research with medical care, only to the extent that the research is justified by its potential prophylactic, diagnostic or therapeutic value. When medical research is combined with medical care, additional standards apply to protect the patients who are research subjects.

29. The benefits, risks, burdens and effectiveness of a new method should be tested against those of the best current prophylactic, diagnostic, and therapeutic methods. This does not exclude the use of placebo, or no treatment, in studies where no proven prophylactic, diagnostic or therapeutic method exists.

30. At the conclusion of the study, every patient entered into the study should be assured of access to the best proven prophylactic, diagnostic and therapeutic methods identified by the study.

31. The physician should fully inform the patient which aspects of the care are related to the research. The refusal of a patient to participate in a study must never interfere with the patient-physician relationship.

32. In the treatment of a patient, where proven prophylactic, diagnostic and therapeutic methods do not exist or have been ineffective, the physician, with informed consent from the patient, must be free to use unproven or new prophylactic, diagnostic and therapeutic measures, if in the physician's judgement it offers hope of saving life, re-establishing health or alleviating suffering. Where possible, these measures should be made the object of research, designed to evaluate their safety and efficacy. In all cases, new information should be recorded and, where appropriate, published. The other relevant guidelines of this Declaration should be followed.

Note: Note of clarification on paragraph 29 of the WMA Declaration of Helsinki
The WMA hereby reaffirms its position that extreme care must be taken in making use of a placebo-controlled trial and that in general this methodology should only be used in the absence of existing proven therapy. However, a placebo-controlled trial may be ethically acceptable, even if proven therapy is available, under the following circumstances:

- Where for compelling and scientifically sound methodological reasons its use is necessary to determine the efficacy or safety of a prophylactic, diagnostic or therapeutic method; or
- Where a prophylactic, diagnostic or therapeutic method is being investigated for a minor condition and the patients who receive placebo will not be subject to any additional risk of serious or irreversible harm.

All other provisions of the Declaration of Helsinki must be adhered to, especially the need for appropriate ethical and scientific review.

Note: Note of clarification on paragraph 30 of the WMA Declaration of Helsinki
The WMA hereby reaffirms its position that it is necessary during the study planning process to identify post-trial access by study participants to prophylactic, diagnostic and therapeutic procedures identified as beneficial in the study or access to other appropriate care. Post-trial access arrangements or other care must be described in the study protocol so the ethical review committee may consider such arrangements during its review.

Appendix 6

The (US) Belmont Report 1979

The Belmont Report
Office of the Secretary

Ethical Principles and Guidelines for the Protection of Human Subjects of Research

The National Commission for the Protection of Human Subjects of Biomedical and Behavioral Research

April 18, 1979

AGENCY: Department of Health, Education, and Welfare.

ACTION: Notice of Report for Public Comment.

SUMMARY: On July 12, 1974, the National Research Act (Pub. L. 93-348) was signed into law, thereby creating the National Commission for the Protection of Human Subjects of Biomedical and Behavioral Research. One of the charges to the Commission was to identify the basic ethical principles that should underlie the conduct of biomedical and behavioral research involving human subjects and to develop guidelines which should be followed to assure that such research is conducted in accordance with those principles. In carrying out the above, the Commission was directed to consider: **(i)** the boundaries between biomedical and behavioral research and the accepted and routine practice of medicine, **(ii)** the role of assessment of risk-benefit criteria in the determination of the appropriateness of research involving human subjects, **(iii)** appropriate guidelines for the selection of human subjects for participation in such research and **(iv)** the nature and definition of informed consent in various research settings.

The Belmont Report attempts to summarize the basic ethical principles identified by the Commission in the course of its deliberations. It is the outgrowth of an intensive four-day period of discussions that were held in February 1976 at the Smithsonian Institution's Belmont Conference Center supplemented by the monthly deliberations of the Commission that were held over a period of nearly four years. It is a statement of basic ethical principles and guidelines that should assist in resolving the ethical problems that surround the conduct of research with human subjects. By publishing the Report in the Federal Register, and providing reprints upon request, the Secretary intends that it may be made readily available to scientists, members of Institutional Review Boards, and Federal employees. The two-volume Appendix, containing the lengthy reports of experts and specialists who assisted the Commission in fulfilling this part of its charge, is available as DHEW Publication No. (OS) 78-0013 and No. (OS) 78-0014, for sale by the Superintendent of Documents, U.S. Government Printing Office, Washington, D.C. 20402.

Unlike most other reports of the Commission, the Belmont Report does not make specific recommendations for administrative action by the Secretary of Health, Education, and Welfare. Rather, the Commission recommended that the Belmont Report be adopted in its entirety, as a statement of the Department's policy. The Department requests public comment on this recommendation.

National Commission for the Protection of Human Subjects of Biomedical and Behavioral Research

Members of the Commission

Kenneth John Ryan, M.D., Chairman, Chief of Staff, Boston Hospital for Women.

Joseph V. Brady, Ph.D., Professor of Behavioral Biology, Johns Hopkins University.

Robert E. Cooke, M.D., President, Medical College of Pennsylvania.

Dorothy I. Height, President, National Council of Negro Women, Inc.

Albert R. Jonsen, Ph.D., Associate Professor of Bioethics, University of California at San Francisco.

Patricia King, J.D., Associate Professor of Law, Georgetown University Law Center.

Karen Lebacqz, Ph.D., Associate Professor of Christian Ethics, Pacific School of Religion.

*** David W. Louisell, J.D., Professor of Law, University of California at Berkeley.

Donald W. Seldin, M.D., Professor and Chairman, Department of Internal Medicine, University of Texas at Dallas.

***Eliot Stellar, Ph.D., Provost of the University and Professor of Physiological Psychology, University of Pennsylvania.

*** Robert H. Turtle, LL.B., Attorney, VomBaur, Coburn, Simmons & Turtle, Washington, D.C.

*** Deceased.

Table of Contents

Ethical Principles and Guidelines for Research Involving Human Subjects

A.   Boundaries Between Practice and Research

B.   Basic Ethical Principles

    1. Respect for Persons

    2. Beneficence

    3. Justice

C.   Applications

    1. Informed Consent

    2. Assessment of Risks and Benefits

    3. Selection of Subjects

Ethical Principles and Guidelines for Research Involving Human Subjects

Scientific research has produced substantial social benefits. It has also posed some troubling ethical questions. Public attention was drawn to these questions by reported abuses of human subjects in biomedical experiments, especially during the Second World War. During the Nuremberg War Crime Trials, the Nuremberg code was drafted as a set of standards for judging physicians and scientists who had conducted biomedical experiments on concentration camp prisoners. This code became the prototype of many later codes[1] intended to assure that research involving human subjects would be carried out in an ethical manner.

The codes consist of rules, some general, others specific, that guide the investigators or the reviewers of research in their work. Such rules often are inadequate to cover complex situations; at times they come into conflict, and they are frequently difficult to interpret or apply. Broader ethical principles will provide a basis on which specific rules may be formulated, criticized and interpreted.

Three principles, or general prescriptive judgments, that are relevant to research involving human subjects are identified in this statement. Other principles may also be relevant. These three are comprehensive, however, and are stated at a level of generalization that should assist scientists, subjects, reviewers and interested citizens to understand the ethical issues inherent in research involving human subjects. These principles cannot always be applied so as to resolve beyond dispute particular ethical problems. The objective is to provide an analytical framework that will guide the resolution of ethical problems arising from research involving human subjects.

This statement consists of a distinction between research and practice, a discussion of the three basic ethical principles, and remarks about the application of these principles.

Part A: Boundaries Between Practice and Research

A.   Boundaries Between Practice and Research

It is important to distinguish between biomedical and behavioral research, on the one hand, and the practice of accepted therapy on the other, in order to know what activities ought to undergo review for the protection of human subjects of research. The distinction between research and practice is blurred partly because both often occur together (as in research designed to evaluate a therapy) and partly because notable departures from standard practice are often called "experimental" when the terms "experimental" and "research" are not carefully defined.

For the most part, the term "practice" refers to interventions that are designed solely to enhance the well-being of an individual patient or client and that have a reasonable expectation of success. The purpose of medical or behavioral practice is to provide diagnosis, preventive treatment or therapy to particular individuals.[2] By contrast, the term "research" designates an activity designed to test a hypothesis, permit conclusions to be drawn, and thereby to develop or contribute to generalizable knowledge (expressed, for example, in theories, principles, and statements of relationships). Research is usually described in a formal protocol that sets forth an objective and a set of procedures designed to reach that objective.

When a clinician departs in a significant way from standard or accepted practice, the innovation does not, in and of itself, constitute research. The fact that a procedure is "experimental," in the sense of new, untested or different, does not automatically place it in the category of research. Radically new procedures of this description should, however, be made the object of formal research at an early stage in order to determine whether they are safe and effective. Thus, it is the responsibility of medical practice committees, for example, to insist that a major innovation be incorporated into a formal research project.[3]

Research and practice may be carried on together when research is designed to evaluate the safety and efficacy of a therapy. This need not cause any confusion regarding whether or not the activity requires review; the general rule is that if there is any element of research in an activity, that activity should undergo review for the protection of human subjects.

Part B: Basic Ethical Principles

B.   Basic Ethical Principles

The expression "basic ethical principles" refers to those general judgments that serve as a basic justification for the many particular ethical prescriptions and evaluations of human actions. Three basic principles, among those generally accepted in our cultural tradition, are particularly relevant to the ethics of research involving human subjects: the principles of respect of persons, beneficence and justice.

1.   Respect for Persons. Respect for persons incorporates at least two ethical convictions: first, that individuals should be treated as autonomous agents, and second, that persons with diminished autonomy are entitled to protection. The principle of respect for persons thus divides into two separate moral requirements: the requirement to acknowledge autonomy and the requirement to protect those with diminished autonomy.

An autonomous person is an individual capable of deliberation about personal goals and of acting under the direction of such deliberation. To respect autonomy is to give weight to autonomous persons' considered opinions and choices while refraining from obstructing their actions unless they are clearly detrimental to others. To show lack of respect for an autonomous agent is to repudiate that person's considered judgments, to deny an individual the freedom to act on those considered judgments, or to withhold information necessary to make a considered judgment, when there are no compelling reasons to do so.

However, not every human being is capable of self-determination. The capacity for self-determination matures during an individual's life, and some individuals lose this capacity wholly or in part because of illness, mental disability, or circumstances that severely restrict liberty. Respect for the immature and the incapacitated may require protecting them as they mature or while they are incapacitated.

Some persons are in need of extensive protection, even to the point of excluding them from activities which may harm them; other persons require little protection beyond making sure they undertake activities freely and with awareness of possible adverse consequence. The extent of protection afforded should depend upon the risk of harm and the likelihood of benefit. The judgment that any individual lacks autonomy should be periodically reevaluated and will vary in different situations.

In most cases of research involving human subjects, respect for persons demands that subjects enter into the research voluntarily and with adequate information. In some situations, however, application of the principle is not obvious. The involvement of prisoners as subjects of research provides an instructive example. On the one hand, it would seem that the principle of respect for persons requires that prisoners not be deprived of the opportunity to volunteer for research. On the other hand, under prison conditions they may be subtly coerced or unduly influenced to engage in research activities for which they would not otherwise volunteer. Respect for persons would then dictate that prisoners be protected. Whether to allow prisoners to "volunteer" or to "protect" them presents a dilemma. Respecting persons, in most hard cases, is often a matter of balancing competing claims urged by the principle of respect itself.

2. Beneficence. Persons are treated in an ethical manner not only by respecting their decisions and protecting them from harm, but also by making efforts to secure their well-being. Such treatment falls under the principle of beneficence. The term "beneficence" is often understood to cover acts of kindness or charity that go beyond strict obligation. In this document, beneficence is understood in a stronger sense, as an obligation. Two general rules have been formulated as complementary expressions of beneficent actions in this sense: (1) do not harm and (2) maximize possible benefits and minimize possible harms.

The Hippocratic maxim "do no harm" has long been a fundamental principle of medical ethics. Claude Bernard extended it to the realm of research, saying that one should not injure one person regardless of the benefits that might come to others. However, even avoiding harm requires learning what is harmful; and, in the process of obtaining this information, persons may be exposed to risk of harm. Further, the Hippocratic Oath requires physicians to benefit their patients "according to their best judgment." Learning what will in fact benefit may require exposing persons to risk. The problem posed by these imperatives is to decide when it is justifiable to seek certain benefits despite the risks involved, and when the benefits should be foregone because of the risks.

The obligations of beneficence affect both individual investigators and society at large, because they extend both to particular research projects and to the entire enterprise of research. In the case of particular projects, investigators and members of their institutions are obliged to give forethought to the maximization of benefits and the reduction of risk that might occur from the research investigation. In the case of scientific research in general, members of the larger society are obliged to recognize the longer term benefits and risks that may result from the improvement of knowledge and from the development of novel medical, psychotherapeutic, and social procedures.

The principle of beneficence often occupies a well-defined justifying role in many areas of research involving human subjects. An example is found in research involving children. Effective ways of treating childhood diseases and fostering healthy development are benefits that serve to justify research involving children – even when individual research subjects are not direct beneficiaries. Research also makes it possible to avoid the harm that may result from the application of previously accepted routine practices that on closer investigation turn out to be dangerous. But the role of the principle of beneficence is not always so unambiguous. A difficult ethical problem remains, for example, about research that presents more than minimal risk without immediate prospect of direct benefit to the children involved. Some have argued that such research is inadmissible, while others have pointed out that this limit would rule out much research promising great benefit to children in the future. Here again, as with all hard cases, the different claims covered by the principle of beneficence may come into conflict and force difficult choices.

3. Justice. Who ought to receive the benefits of research and bear its burdens? This is a question of justice, in the sense of "fairness in distribution" or "what is deserved." An injustice occurs when some benefit to which a person is entitled is denied without good reason or when some burden is imposed unduly. Another way of conceiving the principle of justice is that equals ought to be treated equally. However, this statement requires explication. Who is equal and who is unequal? What considerations justify departure from equal distribution? Almost all commentators allow that distinctions based on experience, age, deprivation, competence, merit and position do sometimes constitute criteria justifying differential treatment for certain purposes. It is necessary, then, to explain in what respects people should be treated equally. There are several widely accepted formulations of just ways to distribute burdens and benefits. Each formulation mentions some relevant property on the basis of which burdens and benefits should be distributed. These formulations are (1) to each person an equal share, (2) to each person according to individual need, (3) to each person according to individual effort, (4) to each person according to societal contribution, and (5) to each person according to merit.

Questions of justice have long been associated with social practices such as punishment, taxation and political representation. Until recently these questions have not generally been associated with scientific research. However, they are foreshadowed even in the earliest reflections on the ethics of research involving human subjects. For example, during the 19th and early 20th centuries the burdens of serving as research subjects fell largely upon poor ward patients, while the benefits of improved medical care flowed primarily to private patients. Subsequently, the exploitation of unwilling prisoners as research subjects in Nazi concentration camps was condemned as a particularly flagrant injustice. In this country, in the 1940's, the Tuskegee syphilis study used disadvantaged, rural black men to study the untreated course of a disease that is by no means confined to that population. These subjects were deprived of demonstrably effective treatment in order not to interrupt the project, long after such treatment became generally available.

Against this historical background, it can be seen how conceptions of justice are relevant to research involving human subjects. For example, the selection of research subjects needs to be scrutinized in order to determine whether some classes (e.g., welfare patients, particular racial and ethnic minorities, or persons confined to institutions) are being systematically selected simply because of their easy availability, their compromised position, or their manipulability, rather than for reasons directly related to the problem being studied. Finally, whenever research supported by public funds leads to the development of therapeutic devices and procedures, justice demands both that these not provide advantages only to those who can afford them and that such research should not unduly involve persons from groups unlikely to be among the beneficiaries of subsequent applications of the research.

Part C: Applications

C.   Applications

Applications of the general principles to the conduct of research lead to consideration of the following requirements: informed consent, risk/benefit assessment, and the selection of subjects of research.

1.   Informed Consent. Respect for persons requires that subjects, to the degree that they are capable, be given the opportunity to choose what shall or shall not happen to them. This opportunity is provided when adequate standards for informed consent are satisfied.

While the importance of informed consent is unquestioned, controversy prevails over the nature and possibility of an informed consent. Nonetheless, there is widespread agreement that the consent process can be analyzed as containing three elements: information, comprehension and voluntariness.

Information. Most codes of research establish specific items for disclosure intended to assure that subjects are given sufficient information. These items generally include: the research procedure, their purposes, risks and anticipated benefits, alternative procedures (where therapy is involved), and a statement offering the subject the opportunity to ask questions and to withdraw at any time from the research. Additional items have been proposed, including how subjects are selected, the person responsible for the research, etc.

However, a simple listing of items does not answer the question of what the standard should be for judging how much and what sort of information should be provided. One standard frequently invoked in medical practice, namely the information commonly provided by practitioners in the field or in the locale, is inadequate since research takes place precisely when a common understanding does not exist. Another standard, currently popular in malpractice law, requires the practitioner to reveal the information that reasonable persons would wish to know in order to make a decision regarding their care. This, too, seems insufficient since the research subject, being in essence a volunteer, may wish to know considerably more about risks gratuitously undertaken than do patients who deliver themselves into the hand of a clinician for needed care. It may be that a standard of "the reasonable volunteer" should be proposed: the extent and nature of information should be such that persons, knowing that the procedure is neither necessary for their care nor perhaps fully understood, can decide whether they wish to participate in the furthering of knowledge. Even when some direct benefit to them is anticipated, the subjects should understand clearly the range of risk and the voluntary nature of participation.

A special problem of consent arises where informing subjects of some pertinent aspect of the research is likely to impair the validity of the research. In many cases, it is sufficient to indicate to subjects that they are being invited to participate in research of which some features will not be revealed until the research is concluded. In all cases of research involving incomplete disclosure, such research is justified only if it is clear that (1) incomplete disclosure is truly necessary to accomplish the goals of the research, (2) there are no undisclosed risks to subjects that are more than minimal, and (3) there is an adequate plan for debriefing subjects, when appropriate, and for dissemination of research results to them. Information about risks should never be withheld for the purpose of eliciting the cooperation of subjects, and truthful answers should always be given to direct questions about the research. Care should be taken to distinguish cases in which disclosure would destroy or invalidate the research from cases in which disclosure would simply inconvenience the investigator.

Comprehension. The manner and context in which information is conveyed is as important as the information itself. For example, presenting information in a disorganized and rapid fashion, allowing too little time for consideration or curtailing opportunities for questioning, all may adversely affect a subject's ability to make an informed choice.

Because the subject's ability to understand is a function of intelligence, rationality, maturity and language, it is necessary to adapt the presentation of the information to the subject's capacities. Investigators are responsible for ascertaining that the subject has comprehended the information.

While there is always an obligation to ascertain that the information about risk to subjects is complete and adequately comprehended, when the risks are more serious, that obligation increases. On occasion, it may be suitable to give some oral or written tests of comprehension.

Special provision may need to be made when comprehension is severely limited – for example, by conditions of immaturity or mental disability. Each class of subjects that one might consider as incompetent (e.g., infants and young children, mentally disabled patients, the terminally ill and the comatose) should be considered on its own terms. Even for these persons, however, respect requires giving them the opportunity to choose to the extent they are able, whether or not to participate in research. The objections of these subjects to involvement should be honored, unless the research entails providing them a therapy unavailable elsewhere. Respect for persons also requires seeking the permission of other parties in order to protect the subjects from harm. Such persons are thus respected both by acknowledging their own wishes and by the use of third parties to protect them from harm.

The third parties chosen should be those who are most likely to understand the incompetent subject's situation and to act in that person's best interest. The person authorized to act on behalf of the subject should be given an opportunity to observe the research as it proceeds in order to be able to withdraw the subject from the research, if such action appears in the subject's best interest.

Voluntariness. An agreement to participate in research constitutes a valid consent only if voluntarily given. This element of informed consent requires conditions free of coercion and undue influence. Coercion occurs when an overt threat of harm is intentionally presented by one person to another in order to obtain compliance. Undue influence, by contrast, occurs through an offer of an excessive, unwarranted, inappropriate or improper reward or other overture in order to obtain compliance. Also, inducements that would ordinarily be acceptable may become undue influences if the subject is especially vulnerable.

Unjustifiable pressures usually occur when persons in positions of authority or commanding influence – especially where possible sanctions are involved – urge a course of action for a subject. A continuum of such influencing factors exists, however, and it is impossible to state precisely where justifiable persuasion ends and undue influence begins. But undue influence would include actions such as manipulating a person's choice through the controlling influence of a close relative and threatening to withdraw health services to which an individual would otherwise be entitled.

2.   Assessment of Risks and Benefits. The assessment of risks and benefits requires a careful arrayal of relevant data, including, in some cases, alternative ways of obtaining the benefits sought in the research. Thus, the assessment presents both an opportunity and a responsibility to gather systematic and comprehensive information about proposed research. For the investigator, it is a means to examine whether the proposed research is properly designed. For a review committee, it is a method for determining whether the risks that will be presented to subjects are justified. For prospective subjects, the assessment will assist the determination whether or not to participate.

The Nature and Scope of Risks and Benefits. The requirement that research be justified on the basis of a favorable risk/benefit assessment bears a close relation to the principle of beneficence, just as the moral requirement that informed consent be obtained is derived primarily from the principle of respect for persons. The term "risk" refers to a possibility that harm may occur.

However, when expressions such as "small risk" or "high risk" are used, they usually refer (often ambiguously) both to the chance (probability) of experiencing a harm and the severity (magnitude) of the envisioned harm.

The term "benefit" is used in the research context to refer to something of positive value related to health or welfare. Unlike "risk," "benefit" is not a term that expresses probabilities. Risk is properly contrasted to probability of benefits, and benefits are properly contrasted with harms rather than risks of harm. Accordingly, so-called risk/benefit assessments are concerned with the probabilities and magnitudes of possible harm and anticipated benefits. Many kinds of possible harms and benefits need to be taken into account. There are, for example, risks of psychological harm, physical harm, legal harm, social harm and economic harm and the corresponding benefits. While the most likely types of harms to research subjects are those of psychological or physical pain or injury, other possible kinds should not be overlooked.

Risks and benefits of research may affect the individual subjects, the families of the individual subjects, and society at large (or special groups of subjects in society). Previous codes and Federal regulations have required that risks to subjects be outweighed by the sum of both the anticipated benefit to the subject, if any, and the anticipated benefit to society in the form of knowledge to be gained from the research. In balancing these different elements, the risks and benefits affecting the immediate research subject will normally carry special weight. On the other hand, interests other than those of the subject may on some occasions be sufficient by themselves to justify the risks involved in the research, so long as the subjects' rights have been protected. Beneficence thus requires that we protect against risk of harm to subjects and also that we be concerned about the loss of the substantial benefits that might be gained from research.

The Systematic Assessment of Risks and Benefits. It is commonly said that benefits and risks must be "balanced" and shown to be "in a favorable ratio." The metaphorical character of these terms draws attention to the difficulty of making precise judgments. Only on rare occasions will quantitative techniques be available for the scrutiny of research protocols. However, the idea of systematic, nonarbitrary analysis of risks and benefits should be emulated insofar as possible. This ideal requires those making decisions about the justifiability of research to be thorough in the accumulation and assessment of information about all aspects of the research, and to consider alternatives systematically. This procedure renders the assessment of research more rigorous and precise, while making communication between review board members and investigators less subject to misinterpretation, misinformation and conflicting judgments. Thus, there should first be a determination of the validity of the presuppositions of the research; then the nature, probability and magnitude of risk should be distinguished with as much clarity as possible. The method of ascertaining risks should be explicit, especially where there is no alternative to the use of such vague categories as small or slight risk. It should also be determined whether an investigator's estimates of the probability of harm or benefits are reasonable, as judged by known facts or other available studies.

Finally, assessment of the justifiability of research should reflect at least the following considerations: (i) Brutal or inhumane treatment of human subjects is never morally justified. (ii) Risks should be reduced to those necessary to achieve the research objective. It should be determined whether it is in fact necessary to use human subjects at all. Risk can perhaps never be entirely eliminated, but it can often be reduced by careful attention to alternative procedures. (iii) When research involves significant risk of serious impairment, review committees should be extraordinarily insistent on the justification of the risk (looking usually to the likelihood of benefit to the subject – or, in some rare cases, to the manifest voluntariness of the participation). (iv) When vulnerable populations are involved in research, the appropriateness of involving them should itself be demonstrated. A number of variables go into such judgments, including the nature and degree of risk, the condition of the particular population involved, and the nature and level of the anticipated benefits. (v) Relevant risks and benefits must be thoroughly arrayed in documents and procedures used in the informed consent process.

3.   Selection of Subjects. Just as the principle of respect for persons finds expression in the requirements for consent, and the principle of beneficence in risk/benefit assessment, the principle of justice gives rise to moral requirements that there be fair procedures and outcomes in the selection of research subjects.

Justice is relevant to the selection of subjects of research at two levels: the social and the individual. Individual justice in the selection of subjects would require that researchers exhibit fairness: thus, they should not offer potentially beneficial research only to some patients who are in their favor or select only "undesirable" persons for risky research. Social justice requires that distinction be drawn between classes of subjects that ought, and ought not, to participate in any particular kind of research, based on the ability of members of that class to bear burdens and on the appropriateness of placing further burdens on already burdened persons. Thus, it can be considered a matter of social justice that there is an order of preference in the selection of classes of subjects (e.g., adults before children) and that some classes of potential subjects (e.g., the institutionalized mentally infirm or prisoners) may be involved as research subjects, if at all, only on certain conditions.

Injustice may appear in the selection of subjects, even if individual subjects are selected fairly by investigators and treated fairly in the course of research. Thus injustice arises from social, racial, sexual and cultural biases institutionalized in society. Thus, even if individual researchers are treating their research subjects fairly, and even if IRBs are taking care to assure that subjects are selected fairly within a particular institution, unjust social patterns may nevertheless appear in the overall distribution of the burdens and benefits of research. Although individual institutions or investigators may not be able to resolve a problem that is pervasive in their social setting, they can consider distributive justice in selecting research subjects.

Some populations, especially institutionalized ones, are already burdened in many ways by their infirmities and environments. When research is proposed that involves risks and does not include a therapeutic component, other less burdened classes of persons should be called upon first to accept these risks of research, except where the research is directly related to the specific conditions of the class involved. Also, even though public funds for research may often flow in the same directions as public funds for health care, it seems unfair that populations dependent on public health care constitute a pool of preferred research subjects if more advantaged populations are likely to be the recipients of the benefits.

One special instance of injustice results from the involvement of vulnerable subjects. Certain groups, such as racial minorities, the economically disadvantaged, the very sick, and the institutionalized may continually be sought as research subjects, owing to their ready availability in settings where research is conducted. Given their dependent status and their frequently compromised capacity for free consent, they should be protected against the danger of being involved in research solely for administrative convenience, or because they are easy to manipulate as a result of their illness or socioeconomic condition.

Notes

1. Since 1945, various codes for the proper and responsible conduct of human experimentation in medical research have been adopted by different organizations. The best known of these codes are the Nuremberg Code of 1947, the Helsinki Declaration of 1964 (revised in 1975), and the 1971 Guidelines (codified into Federal Regulations in 1974) issued by the U.S. Department of Health, Education, and Welfare. Codes for the conduct of social and behavioral research have also been adopted, the best known being that of the American Psychological Association, published in 1973.

2. Although practice usually involves interventions designed solely to enhance the well-being of a particular individual, interventions are sometimes applied to one individual for the enhancement of the well-being of another (e.g., blood donation, skin grafts, organ transplants) or an intervention may have the dual purpose of enhancing the well-being of a particular individual, and, at the same time, providing some benefit to others (e.g., vaccination, which protects both the person who is vaccinated and society generally). The fact that some forms of practice have elements other than immediate benefit to the individual receiving an intervention, however, should not confuse the general distinction between research and practice. Even when a procedure applied in practice may benefit some other person, it remains an intervention designed to enhance the well-being of a particular individual or groups of individuals; thus, it is practice and need not be reviewed as research.

3. Because the problems related to social experimentation may differ substantially from those of biomedical and behavioral research, the Commission specifically declines to make any policy determination regarding such research at this time. Rather, the Commission believes that the problem ought to be addressed by one of its successor bodies.

National Institutes of Health
Bethesda, Maryland 20892

References

1. *Medical Negligence* by Catherine Tay Swee Kian. Times Books International, 2001.

2. Interpretation of the Bolam Test in the Standard of Medical Care: Impact of the Gunapathy Case and Beyond, *Tolley's Journal of Professional Negligence*, Vol. 19, No. 2, 2003 (United Kingdom).

3. Recent Developments in Informed Consent: The Basis of Modern Medical Ethics, *APLAR Journal of Rheumatology*, pages 165–170, December 2005.

4. *Legal Problems in Emergency Medicine* by Alan Montague. Oxford University Press, 1996.

Index